EXPECTING THE GREATEST: THRIVING IN PREGNANCY

EXPECTING THE GREATEST: THRIVING IN PREGNANCY

A PREGNANCY GUIDE

Dr. Shantalasha O. Knowles and Dr. Shamanique S. Bodie-Williams

ISBN-13: 9781975890285
ISBN-10: 1975890280
Library of Congress Control Number: 2017915799
CreateSpace Independent Publishing Platform
North Charleston, South Carolina

We dedicate this book to the author and finisher of our faith, Jesus. He has allowed us to link the facts in medicine with biblical principles. All we do and all we achieve as physicians is through Him.
To all the persons who have contributed positively to our lives and career paths.

Journeys that take time tend to be the ones we remember the most. This journey started in 2008 and to those who made the journey possible thank you. But of note, I thank God for this assignment. Wellington, I thank you for your constant source of love, encouragement and enlightenment. I thank you and love you Lluvia for who you are. Anita, Carlton, Valdez, McCain, and Sharanna, I love and appreciate you more than words can express. Dr. S. Knowles, thank you for journeying with me. Dr. S. Bowe thank you for your ever encouraging voice. Dr. E. Yeomans, Dr. M. Curtis, Dr. R. Gayle, Dr. R. Butler and Mr. R. Fogg, thank you for being mentors that made the difference.
Dr. Shamanique Bodie-Williams

I am grateful for the many people who have impacted me at various points on this literary journey. Thank you God for making impossibilities possible. To my parents; Rodwell and Sybiline, thanks for your unending love and support and for teaching me altruism. To my dear sisters; Tammy, Nevy, Dira and Deria you have been consistent sources of love and my "sounding boards" through it all. Thanks to my entire family who have always supported me. Dr. S. Bodie-Williams, I appreciate your constant encouragement and for taking this path with me. Dr. I. Pratt, Dr. S. Sealy and Dr. D. Francis-Phillips, who have walked with me on my professional medical journey, we made it through teamwork.
Dr. Shantalasha Knowles

TABLE OF CONTENTS

INTRODUCTION

THERE ARE MANY excellent works on the topic of pregnancy and its journey, but none that are geared specifically to persons of Afro-Caribbean descent. When the medical literature is reviewed it would be noted that this group has increased risks of complications and suboptimal outcomes when compared to other groups. Moreover, this group represents the majority of patients that we currently serve in our practice.

Therefore, we wanted to offer a clear voice that could be heard by this group and also other expecting mothers who may not ethnically belong to this group but may have similar concerns and questions. We offer information from an international perspective having training, certifications and professional memberships that are US, European, Caribbean and Asian based. We also offer information that answers common questions and concerns of our patients. Although geared towards expecting mothers, anyone else wanting information on the pregnancy journey will enjoy reading our book. Our voice comes from the heart.

SECTION 1
PREGNANCY PROGRESSION
FROM START TO FINISH

OVERVIEW: CHOOSING YOUR CARE

THE TIME COURSE of pregnancy is measured in weeks and these weeks are separated into distinct periods:

- Weeks 3–8 are called the *embryonic period*.
- Weeks 9 to birth are called the *fetal period*.

The weeks of pregnancy are most commonly divided in three trimesters:

- 0 to 12 weeks: First Trimester
- 13 to 27 weeks: Second Trimester
- 28 to 40 weeks: Third Trimester

Pregnancy can extend to 42 weeks, and this is still considered normal. The age of viability is the gestation at which a baby has the ability to survive outside the womb (although in some cases assistance is needed with treatment). The chance of survival will vary based on the gestation in weeks and the medical support technology available in the country in which you live. The age of viability varies depending on the area in which you live, also. In the Caribbean region, for example, it is 24 weeks in the Bahamas and Jamaica (compared with other countries in the western hemisphere where it is 22 weeks).

It is a common belief that pregnancy is nine months long, but it is actually ten months (40 weeks). Nine months correlates with the time that physicians consider a pregnancy *term*. Term implies that the baby is fully developed and in a normal pregnancy can survive outside of the womb, without having to be attached to mom (well, except maybe only at the breast, but we will talk about breastfeeding later on.)

Once you discover (or suspect) that you are pregnant, you should visit your obstetrician or appropriate healthcare provider. He or she will be able to determine pregnancy through simple tests and an examination and commence your antenatal visits.

In order to determine at what point certain tests should be done in your pregnancy course, monitor the growth of the baby, and decide when you should be delivered, your *estimated due date* (EDD) must be calculated. This can be done by two main methods:

1. The first day of your *last normal menstrual period* (LNMP). This is only accurate in women who have a regular twenty-eight-day menstrual cycle. And even in these women there may be an inability to recall the LNMP, or sometimes the release of the egg from the ovary (ovulation) can vary even in regular cycles. For this reason physicians will most commonly use the second method to determine EDD, as it is most accurate.
2. The measurement of the length of the fetus from the head (crown) to the bottom (rump), known as the *crown-rump length*, by an ultrasound. This is done between 9 and 11 weeks of pregnancy. Once an EDD is determined, it is used throughout the pregnancy.

The EDD does not mean that your baby will be born exactly on that date; most babies are born within two weeks of this date (either before or after). You can track your pregnancy on the many apps available on smartphones. If you are not technologically savvy, your doctor will always keep you abreast of how far you are in the pregnancy at each visit.

Ultrasound can be done at any time during your pregnancy. It uses sound waves that are not harmful to the developing baby when used according to guidelines. It allows the sonographer (the person performing the ultrasound) to see inside the womb by projecting images on a screen. It is an important test to have and can give physicians a wealth of information concerning your pregnancy. It does have its limitations, however, as it cannot detail everything that is happening with your baby. Ultrasounds are done transvaginally by inserting a small part of the machine (the transducer) into the vagina and/or transabdominally by placing the transducer on your abdomen and sliding it around.

HEALTHCARE PROVIDERS: WHO'S WHO

Many different persons take care of pregnant mothers. These range from one primary healthcare provider to a team of healthcare providers.

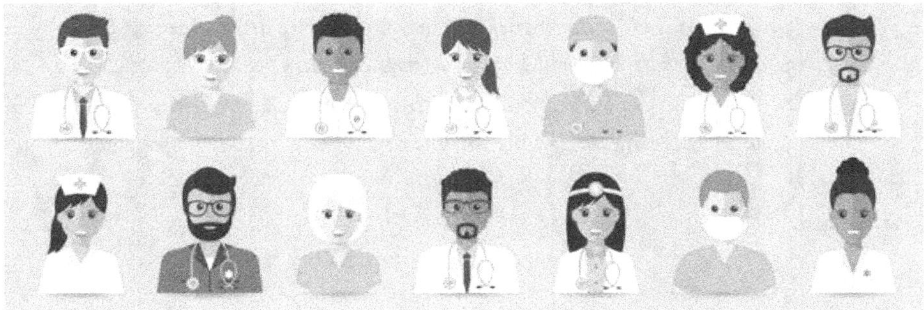

Obstetrician-Gynaecologist (Ob-Gyn):

These are physicians who have been specialist-trained in taking care of the overall health of women from the preconception period to the post-partum period, including family planning and beyond. They are trained in performing surgical procedures involving the mother and fetus. Some ob-gyns are even further trained in maternal-fetal medicine and deal with very high-risk pregnancies that involve various complications to the mother and the fetus.

Family Medicine Physicians

These are physicians that have been trained to take care of the entire family from the infant to the elderly. They also take care of women during the antenatal and postpartum periods. However, if your pregnancy has complications, they will refer you to an ob-gyn.

MIDWIVES

These are persons who have been professionally trained in midwifery (i.e., taking care of the pregnant mother, managing labour and delivery, and dealing with issues in the postpartum period.) In some countries, midwives assume full antenatal care of a pregnant woman. In other countries, they work in conjunction with a physician. Midwives can also be registered nurses first before attaining additional training in midwifery (sometimes called nurse-midwives).

Midwives have been around since the biblical times:

> *"Then the king of Egypt said to the Hebrew midwives…'When you serve as midwife to the Hebrew women and see them on the birthstool, if it is a son, you shall kill him, but if it is a daughter, she shall live.' But the midwives feared God and did not do as the king of Egypt commanded them, but let the male children live."*
>
> —EXODUS 1:15–17 (ESV)

DOULAS

These are persons who are able to provide emotional and physical support to you during your pregnancy and labour and delivery. A doula is not professionally trained to provide medical care or to deliver your baby. A doula does not replace the physician, nurse, or other professionally trained staff.

TYPES OF OBSTETRIC PRACTICES

Community Clinics: Where different doctors trained in women's healthcare are available for you during your pregnancy. Midwives are often apart of community clinic practices.

Solo Practice: When one physician is responsible for your care.

Group Practices: When two or more healthcare providers work together to share in your care. Although only one of these providers may be primarily responsible for your care, they work together to allow you to have constant coverage at all times.

So, what about home births?

Homebirths can be conducive for some mothers as they get to have the entire family (and friends) present and deliver in an environment that they are familiar with. We do not suggest delivery in a place where immediate advanced medical support is not available if needed, however. The time it may take to get to a hospital or such a centre can be the difference between life and death for you and your baby. We suggest that if you live far from medical care or on an island where rapid access to such centres may be difficult that you make sure you are temporarily relocated close enough to get to these centres in a timely manner (especially if you are a high-risk patient or approaching term). Studies have shown babies have two times the risk of dying at a home birth (versus a hospital birth) and three times the risk of having brain injuries or seizures. If you are pregnant with more than one baby, have had a previous caesarean section, or your baby is not head-down first, you should not have a home birth. It is recommended that home births be attended to by at least a certified midwife. A conversation with your healthcare provider on this issue will give you good insight.

C H A P T E R   1

THE FIRST TRIMESTER

PREGNANCY CAN BE a very happy time for Mom, Dad, and rest of the family. Every day there is anticipation as the baby grows. Initially mom may not feel any different, and the growth of the baby cannot be seen outwardly. We want to give you a glimpse into the womb regarding the development of your baby.

WEEKS 1–4

In the first week, there is a process that occurs called *fertilisation* where the sperm meets and joins with the egg (the oocyte). This is not an easy task for the sperm; it must compete for the egg with about two hundred million other sperm. Wow! Isn't that amazing? It is only one sperm, however, that is victorious in this battle.

The cells of this combination divide repeatedly to get larger and form a ball of cells called an embryo. Did you know the sex of your baby is determined at fertilisation? The sperm that is carrying an X produces an XX embryo (female) and the sperm carrying a Y produces an XY embryo (male). The actual genitalia, however, are not seen until much later when the baby is bigger.

Week 1: During the first week, this ball of cells (at this time called the *morula*) makes its journey down the fallopian tubes to the uterus, where it will make its home for the weeks to come. The embryo is very tiny at this stage (and is called the *blastocyst*).

Week 2: During this time, the embryo implants into the lining of the uterus (the *endometrium*). Some women may have spotting of blood around this time that they think is a period; this is referred to as *implantation bleed.*

This can confuse the mother when she is trying to recall when her last period was.

Week 3: Cells of the embryo form small finger-like projections known as *villi* that penetrate deep into the lining of the uterus to form a connecting system to the mother's arteries. The connecting system will later form the afterbirth (the *placenta*). The placenta is very important in pregnancy. It allows nutrients and oxygen to pass to the baby and waste to pass back out to mom. The baby could not live without it. An umbilical cord eventually forms between the baby and mom's blood supply. It is a twisting of two arteries and one vein. It attaches the baby to the placenta (we will talk more about this in chapter 14). The cells of the embryo also begin to produce "the pregnancy hormone," formally known as *human chorionic gonadotropin* (hCG). It is at this time that home pregnancy tests become positive (because of the presence of this hormone). Progesterone and estrogen are also produced, and these tell your ovaries to not release any more eggs; your period also stops. The organs of the baby are beginning to develop as early as week 3 as well.

Week 4: Development of the organs continues, such as the brain structures, nerves, spinal cord, heart, and lungs. Although all these organs are

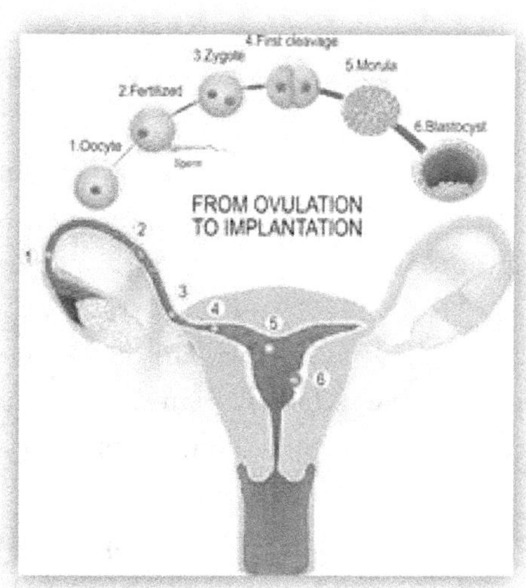

Figure 1. Fertilisation

developing, they are not yet fully functioning. The heart does begin to beat at this time. Your doctor may be able to detect it during an ultrasound exam, but if it is not heard don't worry, not every heartbeat will be picked up this early, even when it is there. Repeating the ultrasound in about two weeks is not uncommon; by this time the heartbeat will definitely be heard. Some mothers describe the sound as "music to their ears." At this time your baby also becomes enveloped in a sac that acts somewhat as a protective barrier, known as the *amniotic sac*. This sac contains a clear fluid (*amniotic fluid*) in which your baby can move about in freely. This sac can be compared to a balloon filled with water.

We are intricately designed by God, our Maker. God said:

"Before I formed you in the womb, I knew you."

—*JEREMIAH 1:5* (ESV)

WEEK 5–8

During this time, the baby continues to grow and develop. The limbs form as tiny appendages that look like paddles and eventually form grooves that allow for the separation of fingers and toes. The gut (or digestive tract) develops. The baby now begins to take a form that is recognizable with a face, ears, nose, eyes, and even eyelids (but they are not open yet). Even though all these exciting changes are taking place, the baby is still very small, only about the size of a grape by week 8. When organs begin to develop, the baby is extremely sensitive to toxins or drugs that may enter the body of the mother or genetic abnormalities, and these can sometimes lead to birth defects.

Women with monthly regular periods will now notice that they have missed a period. This is the time to head on over to your doctor to get a pregnancy test. Some women do this test at home, but it is important to know that even when pregnant, this test can be negative if it is not done at the proper time of day. A test that is truly positive will most commonly be positive when an early morning sample of urine is tested. Your physician can do a blood test if you suspect you may be pregnant but your urine test is negative.

WEEKS 9–12

Well, look at this; you have reached your third month of pregnancy. We know you are still wondering why you can't see your abdomen protruding yet or feel any movement, but don't worry, it is coming shortly. At this point the baby is moving, but it is too minute for you to perceive it.

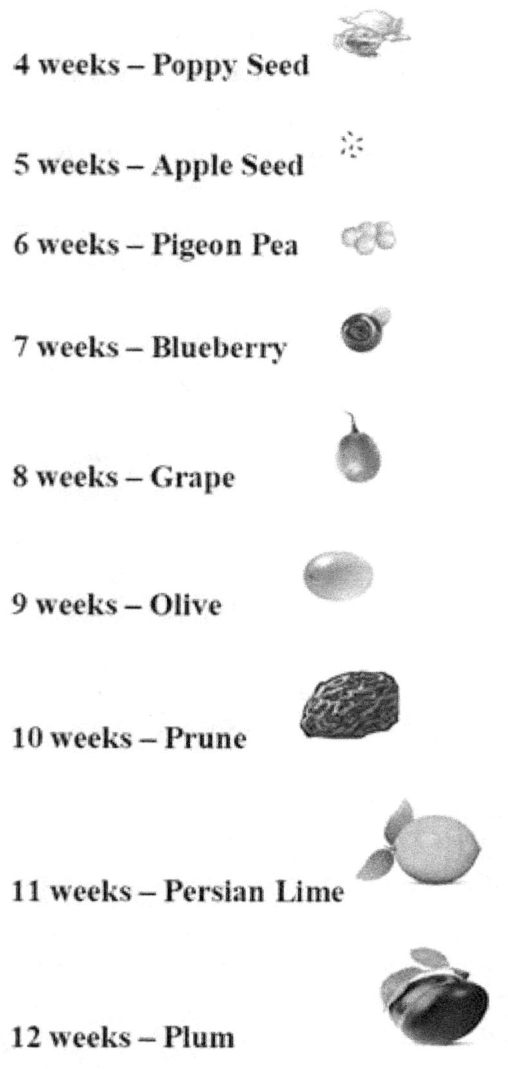

Figure 2. Size of the embryo/fetus in the first trimester

Your baby's sex hormones, estrogen and testosterone, begin to be produced, and bones and teeth start to develop as well (though they are not hard like adult bones as yet, and the teeth have not yet erupted through the gums). The skin is very thin (even thinner than an onion skin) and your baby is the size of a Persian lime.

FIRST TRIMESTER TESTING

Ultrasound: (usually transvaginally) to determine the EDD, the number of babies, if the pregnancy is implanted in the incorrect place (we will talk about an ectopic pregnancy in chapter 30), and if the pregnancy is not a miscarriage.

Screening for Birth Abnormalities: tests that can be performed on the baby to determine if your baby is at risk for certain birth defects. The most common defects include Trisomy 21 (Down's syndrome), Trisomy 18, and neural tube defects (which are abnormalities that can occur along the spinal cord and areas of the brain). They are initially done with a blood test and are then confirmed using chorionic villi sampling or amniocentesis. Some genetic conditions can also be determined with these diagnostic tests when certain hereditary diseases may exist in the family. These samples from the baby are obtained through aspirating a small amount of the tissue from the afterbirth using a needle guided by the ultrasound (chorionic villi sampling) or by aspirating a minimal amount of amniotic fluid from the amniotic sac (amniocentesis).

Antenatal Laboratory Tests: routinely done in every pregnant patient and include the following:

- *Haemoglobin levels* to determine the ability of the red blood cells in your body to deliver oxygen to your baby through the placenta. This level should be greater than or equal to 10 g/dl in a pregnant woman. Haemoglobin also helps to deliver iron to the baby for proper growth. If this level is low, you are anemic and may need additional iron to increase the number.

- *Blood group and rhesus type.* There are four main blood types: A, B, AB, and O. Your rhesus type can be either negative or positive, which refers to a particular protein carried on the blood cells known as the *rhesus antigen*. If your baby carries this protein but you do not (that is, you are rhesus negative) it may result in other proteins in your body attacking the baby's blood cells and leading to anemia in the baby, and if severe it can also cause the baby's heart to fail. If you are rhesus negative you will be given a medication called RhoGAM® to help prevent this in your pregnancy.

- *Sexually transmitted infections test,* to detect such STDs as human immunodeficiency virus (HIV), syphilis, chlamydia, gonorrhoea, and trichomoniasis.

- *Urine testing* for urinary tract infections (which are common in pregnancy and can be treated). Also urine is tested for proteins associated with high blood pressure in pregnancy.

- *Rubella antibody levels* to ensure they are adequate which confirms that you have been vaccinated against rubella or you have had the disease in the past and have mounted an appropriate antibody response to protect you in the future against rubella.

- *Glucose tolerance test* to determine if a pregnant woman is at risk for diabetes during the course of her pregnancy.

- *Papanicolaou smear (Pap smear)* to check for abnormal cells of the cervix (neck of the womb). Pregnancy (or the postpartum period) is a good time to do this screening, as some women may only present to a doctor during pregnancy.

- *Hepatitis B*. This is a waterborne or sexually transmitted infection that can be passed onto the fetus in the womb. If you are found to be positive, treatment will be given to your baby.

- *Group B Streptococcus (GBS)*. This is a bacterium that can live in the vagina or rectum of women and pass onto the baby as it moves through the birth canal during delivery, making the baby very sick. Screening for GBS is done between 35 to 37 weeks.

At every antenatal visit your healthcare provider will measure your weight, take your blood pressure, and test your urine.

BODY CHANGES AND OTHER EXPECTATIONS DURING THE FIRST TRIMESTER

Nutrition/Weight Gain: Often women believe that they are now "eating for two" and should increase the amount of food they eat. This is true, to an extent. It is important that pregnant women eat well, but the intake of calories should not be excessive as this can lead to other complications within the pregnancy such as diabetes. The amount of weight that should be gained is based on your *body mass index* (BMI), which is calculated from your height and weight. This should ideally be your weight just prior to pregnancy. BMI categories are as follows in kg/m^2: underweight (<18.5), normal weight (18.5–24.9), overweight (25–29.9), and obese (>30). Table 1 shows how much weight you should aim to gain in a healthy way depending on what BMI you are starting at.[1]

Table 1

Current BMI	Recommended total weight gain in pounds	How fast weight should be gained in the second and third trimesters (pounds per week)
Underweight	28–40 (12.7-18.1 kg)	1–1.3
Normal weight	25–35 (11.3-15.9 kg)	0.8–1
Overweight	15–25 (6.8-11.3 kg)	0.5–0.7
Obese	11–20 (5-9.1 kg)	0.4–0.6

You may need to consult with a nutritionist during your pregnancy to help you stay on tract, particularly if you are vegetarian or vegan. Your healthcare provider will closely monitor your weight gain and will advise you on steps to take to remain within your weight goals. Weight loss is not wise during pregnancy as strict restriction of calories can lead to learning problems later

---

1 Adapted based on data from the Institutes of Medicine, *Weight Gain During Pregnancy: Reexamining the Guidelines*, Washington, DC: National Academic Press, 2009.

on with your child. An important nutrient at this time in the pregnancy is folic acid. Folic acid is found in dark green leafy vegetables. When it is insufficient in the diet, it can lead to neural tube defects. The daily requirement is 0.4 mg. Many women may not get this in normal meals, so women (even when not pregnant) should take daily multivitamins that include folic acid in this amount at least.

Sleeping and Fatigue: There are two ends of the spectrum when it comes to sleeping during this trimester of pregnancy. Most women will discover that they always feel tired or fatigued. As a result, some are unable to fall asleep or stay asleep at night and others find that they are sleeping all the time. Many pregnancy changes contribute to this often-overwhelming tiredness, including a lower blood pressure, a fall in the haemoglobin level, and a decrease in blood sugar levels. During these times it is comforting to have the Word of God to turn to.

"In peace I will lie down and sleep, for you alone, O LORD,
will keep me safe."

—PSALM 4:8 (NLT)

Sex: Sexual intercourse is safe in pregnancy during this time. Normally during vaginal intercourse the penis may abut the neck of the womb (cervix) and due to the increased blood supply to the cervix, there can be minimal spotting of blood occurring up to a few days after sex. This is usually not ominous, although it may be scary for the pregnant mother. Bleeding occurring at any time during pregnancy should warrant a call or a visit to your healthcare provider to ensure there is not another cause for the bleeding. Sex has not been shown to cause miscarriages or cause harm to the fetus.

Exercise: Mothers often get concerned about "pregnancy fat" so to speak and may want to continue to maintain a regular exercise regime while pregnant. This is quite acceptable at this time. It must be remembered that additional blood supply is required to get to the muscles during exercise and that must be balanced with the growing fetus (who also need blood supply from the mother).

You must never exercise to the point of feeling breathless or like you are about to faint. With this in mind, low-impact aerobic exercises will keep you healthy and may alleviate some of the common symptoms in pregnancy, such as backache and fatigue, while not compromising the fetus in any way. If you were physically active before pregnancy, it is often easy to continue, but don't try to start a rigorous exercise schedule with new activities if you did not exercise prior to pregnancy. Thirty minutes a day on most days of the week is quite sufficient to maintain fitness. Examples of activities that can be carried out include swimming and walking. Drink plenty of water, avoid exercise on uneven surfaces, and avoid exercising on very hot days (as known in the Caribbean, the temperature can soar to the high nineties in the summer months). Before exercising, discuss it with your healthcare provider, so together you can come up with a plan that suits your individual needs and circumstances.

Travel: Travel in the first trimester of pregnancy is generally safe. It is important when taking extended air travel, sea travel or road trips (generally four hours or more) that you intermittently remain mobile. Immobility during travel can lead to the development of blood clots (*deep vein thrombosis*), which most commonly occurs in the calves. Pregnant women are at a greater chance of developing blood clots. The clot can also circulate in the body, making its way to the lungs and resulting in sudden chest pain, shortness of breath, or even death from a condition known as a *pulmonary embolism*. To help prevent this, regularly massage the calves, move the ankles, wear loose-fitting clothing, and remain well hydrated during long trips. On road trips, take several rest stops and walk around for a bit. Symptoms of a deep vein thrombosis and resulting pulmonary embolism can appear hours to even a month after travelling.

Work: Work practice may be discussed with your healthcare provider regarding work policies and to determine if changes in workload are needed.

Home: Household duties may need to be lessened due to the increased fatigue experienced at this time.

Headaches and Dizziness: These tend to become more frequent or first appear at this time. Dizziness can start quite early in pregnancy and is usually due to the changes in the way blood flows through the vessels during pregnancy and the way the body uses food for fuel. This is discussed in more detail in chapter 28.

Heightened Smelling Sense: In pregnancy some women may notice that certain smells and odors cause them to feel upset in the stomach (nauseous). It can also cause vomiting. These smells can range from foods to perfumes.

Nausea and Vomiting: This is usually a fear of many pregnant women. "I hope I don't vomit during my pregnancy" is a line that is all too familiar. But, as with anything that you may fear, always remember God gives us the strength to persevere through anything we are faced with, if we trust Him to do so.

"For God has not given us a spirit of fear and timidity, but of power, love, and self-discipline"

—2 TIMOTHY 1:7 (NLT)

The increase in the hCG hormone, which we spoke about earlier, is the culprit in nausea and vomiting in pregnancy in the first trimester. A heightened sense of smell that occurs in pregnancy can contribute to nausea and vomiting also. Usually after 12 weeks you may no longer have these symptoms (although some people have to endure it up until delivery). Some tips in helping are to eat small, frequent meals (up to six times a day), including crackers as a snack, and avoid spicy or acidic foods. You may find that certain foods, ginger teas, mints, or gums are also helpful with decreasing nausea. When the nausea and vomiting becomes so severe that it leads to dehydration and weight loss, often requiring a visit to the hospital, this is referred to as *hyperemesis gravidarum* (a condition that requires its own moment in time for discussion in chapter 21).

Tender Breasts: Your breasts may begin to become tender to the touch, and this is due to the pregnancy hormones circulating in the body. They act on the breast tissue, preparing it for growth and milk production.

Vaginal Bleeding: Bleeding in pregnancy is never normal; however, it can occur in the first trimester for various reasons. Vessels in the body during pregnancy increase their blood flow, and this includes blood flow to the cervix. Infections of the cervix can cause it to bleed and, as stated earlier, sexual intercourse can also. Bleeding in the first trimester can also be a heralding sign of a pregnancy loss. Unfortunately, in most cases, nothing can be done to prevent a pregnancy loss at this time that has been forewarned with bleeding. If the bleeding stops, this is referred to as a threatened miscarriage, and the pregnancy may continue normally to term.

Constipation: As the level of progesterone increases during pregnancy, it may cause you to experience constipation. Progesterone slows down the movement of the bowel, allowing stools to remain in the rectum longer and making it more difficult to pass stools when it is time to. As the stool sits in the rectum, it also can become harder.

This is a common complaint that you may experience while being pregnant especially if you had problems with constipation before becoming pregnant. Some ways to alleviate this include:

- Increase your intake of water, fruits, vegetables, and fibre. Pace your increase so you do not suffer from gas and bloating.
- Eat protein that is easy to digest, such as eggs and fish, until your bowel movements are soft and regular.
- Try to eat smaller meals in more frequent portions.
- Avoid caffeinated beverages.
- Consider adding a probiotic to your diet.
- Use stool softeners such as docusate sodium (e.g., Colace®, Phillip's Liquid Gel®) for short-term use.
- Consider a time set aside for the bathroom so you will not feel rushed.
- Go to the bathroom when you have the urge and do not delay.
- Exercise regularly (e.g., walking for twenty minutes a day).
- Consider a massage by a massage therapist who specializes in pregnancy massage.
- Use a small amount of coconut or almond oil around the rectum to make the passage of the stool easier.

Natural remedies for constipation include prunes, papaya, natural yogurt, kefir (fermented milk), lacto-fermented pickles, relishes, sauerkraut, molasses, honey, and herbal teas. Avoid mineral oils or laxatives unless under the direction of your physician.

FIRST TRIMESTER CHECKLIST

- ✓ Choose a doctor. This can be any qualified obstetrician with whom you are comfortable. In some settings you may be seen by a group comprising of several physicians and nurses in a clinic in your country.
- ✓ Inform your doctor of any medications you are taking at the first visit.
- ✓ Obtain an ultrasound.
- ✓ Take your antenatal vitamins.
- ✓ Check your health insurance (if this applies to you).
- ✓ Quit smoking.
- ✓ Quit alcoholic intake.
- ✓ Decrease caffeine intake.
- ✓ Budget for your baby.

After reading this chapter, we are sure you may be thinking about how you will adjust to the many changes pregnancy entails. But remember you are not in this journey alone; God is there.

"As one whom his mother comforts, so will I comfort you."

—Isaiah 66:13 (ESV)

C H A P T E R 2

THE SECOND TRIMESTER

ONE TRIMESTER DOWN, two more to go. As a mother, you should be excited as your pregnancy advances. This second trimester is filled with new experiences. You will now start to see some obvious changes in the size of your abdomen, known as "showing" as some cultures refer to the first appearance of a protruding abdomen that can be noticed by others.

WEEKS 13–16

During this time, the placenta continues to develop and it has two parts: the side facing the fetus (which is smooth in contour) and the side facing the inside of the mother's uterus (which is made up of bumpy, bulging areas called *cotyledons*). The placenta now produces hormones like progesterone (that maintains the pregnancy) and human placental lactogen that causes breast development and milk production.

The kidneys in your baby now begin to produce urine. It is this urine from the kidneys that contribute to the amount of amniotic fluid present in the amniotic sac. Drinking excessive water does not cause the fluid in the sac to increase.

In the male fetus, the external (outside) genitalia begin to form to give rise to a penis and the sac in which the testes will be housed (the scrotal sac). In the female, the external genitalia form to give rise to the vagina, lips of the vulva, and clitoris. The external genitalia now start to look distinctly male or female.

"So God created human beings in his own image. In the image
of God he created them; male and female he created them."

—GENESIS 1:27 (NLT)

"He created them male and female, and he blessed them and called them 'human.'"

—GENESIS 5:2 (NLT)

WEEKS 17–20

Testes (in boys) and ovaries (in girls) are formed by this time. The testes begin to descend into the scrotal sac (this decent, however, is not complete until the third trimester). As the genitals are developed, this is an opportune time to see the gender of your baby by ultrasound.

The skin is becoming thicker, and skin glands produce a secretion call *vernix*, which is a sticky white substance that coats the baby's skin until birth. It is waterproof and protects the baby's skin. The skin is also covered with very fine, lightly coloured hair known as *lanugo hair*.

If this is your first pregnancy you will begin to feel your baby's movements during this period. Initially it may feel like a fluttering, and then it will become stronger kicks with time. The baby weighs about half a pound now.

WEEKS 21–24

The gut (digestive system) of the baby begins to produce what is known as the first stool, called *meconium*. It is greenish-black, thick, and pasty and will be passed sometime prior to delivery or just after birth. Do not be alarmed when you see this unusual looking stool in your baby's diaper at the first change.

Ultrasounds done at this time may catch your baby sucking its fingers. He or she goes through cycles of sleeping and being awake, but most time is spent sleeping. The eyes are well developed, but the eyelids remain closed until about 23 to 24 weeks. Your baby weighs about one pound now.

WEEKS 25–28

As growth and development continues, your baby begins to respond to sounds. A loud sound can startle them, and movements are much more obvious. The baby kicks and opens and closes its hands and can even grab onto the umbilical cord. Special skin cells called *melanocytes* secrete *melanin*, which gives the skin its colour. Melanin continues to be produced after birth. Your baby weighs about 1.5 to 2 pounds by 28 weeks.

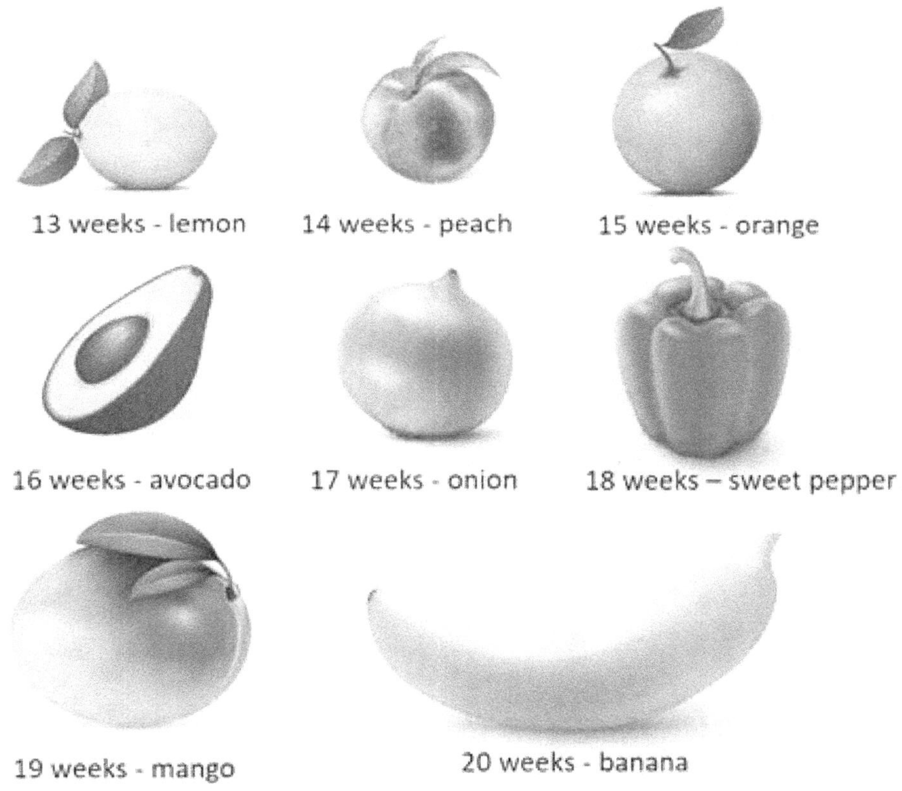

Figure 3. The size of the fetus in the second trimester

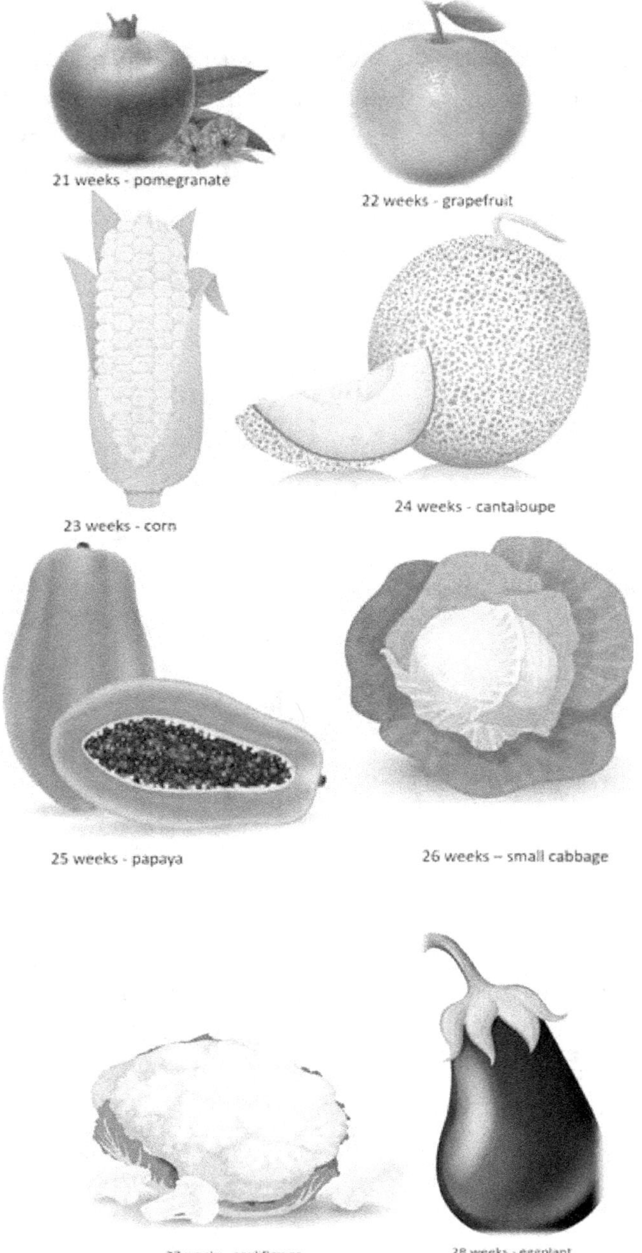

Figure 4. The size of the fetus in the latter half of the second trimester

SECOND TRIMESTER TESTING

Ultrasound: This ultrasound may be the one that is most exciting for the parents as body parts will be much more recognizable to you. Many mothers want to know whether they are having a girl or a boy, and this can be determined at 16 to 20 weeks. But before you go out to decorate the nursery or buy clothes, it is important to know that the accuracy of an ultrasound for gender determination is not 100 percent. Also, if the baby is not in the right position, the healthcare provider may not be able to see the gender. Rarely is the gender of the baby important to your medical care (except with certain genetic conditions). Requesting an ultrasound just for this purpose is not ideal.

Between 18 to 20 weeks is the ideal time to look for fetal abnormalities that might have occurred during the period of organ development in the first trimester. A detailed evaluation is done. As advanced as ultrasound technology is, it is still possible that all abnormalities may not be seen and may be discovered only after birth.

Screening for Birth Abnormalities: The screening test that your healthcare provider will request at this time is called the *quadruple screen*. This is done between 15 and 20 weeks of pregnancy. It is a test that assesses for the likelihood that your baby may be born with any of the more common chromosomal abnormalities, in particular Down's syndrome or neural tube defects. This screen measures the level of four hormones in the body: estriol, maternal serum alpha-fetoprotein, inhibin A, and hCG. A combination of these test results and your age will determine your risk of having a baby with an abnormality as mentioned above.

A positive test result does not absolutely confirm an abnormality nor tell the exact type, which can only be done by amniocentesis, which collects some of the fluid in the amniotic sac and analyzes it by looking at the chromosomes. Amniocentesis is a simple procedure, where an area on the abdomen is cleaned with a special solution and a needle is inserted in the amniotic sac with the guide of a real-time ultrasound image. Although it is a common and simple procedure, complications can occur (rarely), including infection, bleeding, and early "breaking of the waters" (known as *rupture of the membranes*).

Antenatal Laboratory Tests: In the second trimester the only routine blood test that will be offered is a glucose test. In populations where many women have factors that increase their risk for diabetes (e.g., in the Bahamas), this test can be done in the first trimester and, if negative, repeated in the second trimester. When performed in the second trimester, it is done between 24 and 28 weeks of pregnancy. This test and how the results are interpreted are discussed later on in chapter 13.

Antenatal Examinations: Starting around 20 weeks, your healthcare provider will begin to measure your fundal height. This is the distance from the upper border of your pelvic bone (*symphysis pubis*) to the top of your uterus, called the fundus (see figure 5). The fundal height (in centimetres) should correlate with how many weeks pregnant you are. So, if you are 24 weeks your fundal height will be 21 to 27 cm (on average). This fundal height helps to determine how well your baby is growing and will be done at every visit from the second trimester onward.

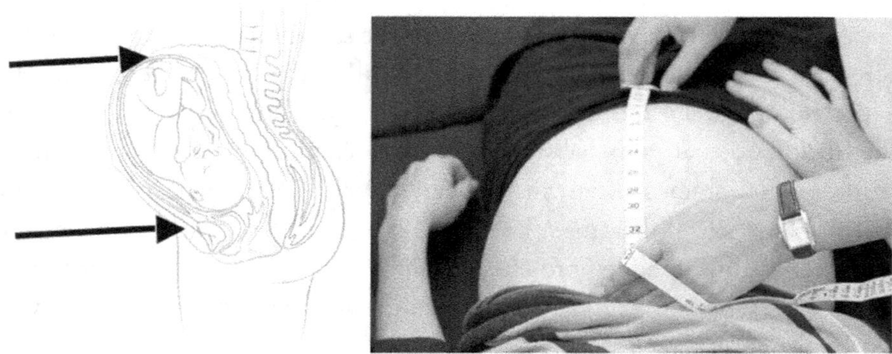

Figure 5. Fundus (top arrow), symphysis pubis (bottom arrow)

BODY CHANGES AND OTHER EXPECTATIONS DURING THE SECOND TRIMESTER

Sleeping: Finding a comfortable position to sleep in may be a task. Although sleeping on your tummy causes no harm to the baby, you may not find it to be conducive to a good night's rest. Side-sleeping is better than back-sleeping in the second trimester. This is because your enlarging uterus can compress some large vessels that are located in the abdomen and pelvis, decreasing the blood flowing to the baby or causing you to become dizzy. Also lying too flat can cause acid reflux as well. However, don't be afraid if you happen to roll onto your back during sleep; the short time spent there is not a problem. Try propping up your pillow(s) and sleeping with a pillow between the legs and ankles, as this will help in keeping the spine straight and may relieve backache through the sleeping hours. Full-length pillows may also be beneficial.

Sex: You can participate in sexual intercourse with your husband straight through the second trimester. As your uterus enlarges, some couples may find it more technically challenging either due to supporting the increasing weight of the uterus or impeding penile penetration. Using alternate positions may help. For example, woman on the top takes the weight off of the uterus that would occur with the missionary position yet facilitates penile penetration. Side by side allows penile entrance from behind. On all fours supports your weight on hands and knees and allows entrance into the vagina from behind. You may experience cramping after sex due to orgasm or, as noted earlier, spotting of blood. Neither of these are concerning, but if cramping persists and bleeding is heavy, you should contact your healthcare provider. Lastly, some women report overwhelming emotions after orgasm and may cry unexpectedly. There is not a clear scientific reason for this, but it may be related to the increasing hormone levels, particularly estrogen.

Travel: Travelling towards the early to mid–second trimester is safe if you have no pregnancy complications. However, as you get closer to the third trimester, long travel is not advised. Check with the airline or cruise line as to what the travel limits are in pregnancy. If you are travelling by car make sure that you wear your seat belt. Move your seat back a little further away from the airbags, but leave them enabled. While travelling, pack an extra supply of your supplements and some antinausea medication. Stay hydrated during your trip.

If you are planning international or even regional travel, it is important to be aware of communicable diseases in the areas you are going to that can affect your baby. Vaccinations are often given to nonpregnant women who are embarking on travel to certain areas (e.g., yellow fever vaccination for travel to

Trinidad), but most of these vaccines are contraindicated in pregnancy. If you are travelling to areas where malaria is present, your physician can prescribe a drug that helps to protect against malaria.

Investigate the healthcare facilities and providers at your selected destination. If an emergency occurs, then you would know where to go. Take some information such as a health summary or ultrasound report from your provider when you travel in the event you have to seek medical care. Check with your healthcare provider before travelling.

Work: Work is still possible during this stage; however, if you work on a job that requires lifting heavy objects, climbing, or standing for many hours, it may be advisable for you to discontinue work or to cut back on your hours. Dizziness, fatigue, and nausea can decrease your productivity at work. Discuss your work duties with your healthcare provider so that you can decide together if you should continue work. Some employers should allow for a switch in work duties while you are pregnant. While at work keep snacks handy, drink plenty fluids, and take naps during your lunch break if you can.

Home: Avoid lifting and moving heavy objects, such as furniture or a laundry basket filled with clothes. As much as possible avoid cleaning with chemical solvents (household cleaners). If you must clean, do it in a well-ventilated area and wear gloves. Care should be taken when mopping and vacuuming the floors.

Exercise: As your weight increases and your abdomen protrudes, you may find that it is more difficult to keep your balance. Exercise should therefore be any activity in which you are safe from falling, for example floor stretches. Contact sports or any high-impact sports or exercises should definitely be avoided. Although swimming is still safe, diving should not be done as it can cause injury to the fetus.

COMMON COMPLAINTS

Increasing Vaginal Discharge: The hormones produced in pregnancy have an effect on normal vaginal secretions causing it to increase. These secretions can be white, tan, or slightly yellow in colour and creamy in consistency, but they should not have an odor. If you notice a bad odor or a fish-like odor, it means an infection is present and you need to be treated by your health-care provider. *Bacterial vaginosis* is a common vaginal infection that causes this fishy odor. A clumpy or cottage cheese–like discharge is seen with yeast infections and can be treated easily; however, this infection tends to recur in pregnancy. It is commonly associated with vaginal itching and redness. The pregnancy hormones cause certain bacteria to overgrow and cause these infections.

Enlarging Breasts: In this trimester, the breast tenderness experienced during the first trimester has usually stopped. Now, however, you may find that you have to make a trip to the underwear store to purchase a larger bra. The breast tissue in the second trimester grows significantly, particularly towards the end. This occurs because the milk glands in the breast (the mammary glands along with its system of ducts that take milk to the nipple) begin to grow in order to ensure a good supply of *colostrum* (first milk) and continuing supply on your baby's demand after birth. Some other changes you may notice is a darkening of the skin around the nipple, known as the *areolar*, and the appearance of "bumps" called *Montgomery tubercles*. These help to lubricate the nipple with oily secretions to keep it supple and protected as your baby breastfeeds. The changes to your breast may seem strange initially, but these changes are normal. You may also notice the veins underneath the skin becoming very visible; this is due to the increase in blood flow to the breast.

Abdominal Cramps: These can be similar in intensity and character like mild period pain or they can become more severe running towards the groin and legs due to stretching of rope-like structures (called *ligaments*) that hold the uterus in place. These pains tend to resolve over time or, if unable to be tolerated, analgesics can be taken.

Towards the end of the second trimester you may also experience a tightening and relaxing sensation of the uterus that may be painless or cause mild to moderate pain, this is known as *Braxton-Hicks contractions*. You can think of these contractions as getting you ready for the real thing. They may occur on and off for several minutes or may last much longer and become more frequent the closer you get to term. Consult your healthcare provider if the pains are unrelenting and increasing in intensity or frequency, as this may signal that preterm labour is ensuing.

Lower Backache: There is much strain on the back as pregnancy advances. The enlarging uterus causes the spine to take an inward curvature known as *lordosis,* and this can contribute to backache. Here are some tips for preventing or relieving backache:

- Wear flat shoes (yes, we know, it may not look as cute, but it will spare you pain and also the possibility of losing your balance and falling).
- Prevent standing for long periods of time.
- Stoop to pick up objects, instead of bending over.
- Carry a cushion to support your back when sitting for a long time.

Numbness in the Hands: This can slow you down on working with your hands and is sometimes associated with pain. Numbness tends to be more severe at nighttime, which can disturb sleep or be present on waking up. The body retains more fluids in the soft tissues and when this fluid accumulates around the wrist, it compresses a nerve that runs down the middle of the arm to the wrist and fingers. This compression leads to numbness, which in this case is called *carpal tunnel syndrome.*

Legs and Feet Swelling: So, you went and pulled out your favorite pair of shoes, and they don't fit! Swollen feet and legs can be alarming but are usually not a problem and occur in about 80 percent of pregnant women. The change in the way the blood circulates through the body causes blood to move more slowly from the legs, and fluid can accumulate in the tissues just below the skin, leading to swollen legs. When the fluid is excessive, it can cause a sensation of tightness in the leg and mild pain. Calf pain, however, should not be ignored, as this could be a sign of something more dangerous, like a deep vein thrombosis. Keep your feet elevated as much as possible in the daytime.

Haemorrhoids: This is a common condition that may occur in pregnancy. It happens when the blood vessels to the rectum, the external haemorrhoidal veins, become varicose, which causes itching burning and swelling in the back passage. It may also cause pain with bowel movements and blood in the stool. There are other possible causes of blood in the stool, and you should see your healthcare provider so they can make the diagnosis and recommended treatment.

Some things that you can do to prevent haemorrhoids include increasing the fibre in your diet (with fruits, vegetables, and whole grains), increasing your fluid intake, taking stool softeners, bathing with warm water, and using local ointments or suppositories.

There is a good chance that with these conservative measures your symptoms will improve, and most will resolve after you give birth. For those that do not resolve, there are surgical options available postdelivery.

Stretch Marks: This is something that many pregnant women dread. As your uterus grows, it puts tremendous strain on your skin, causing a breakdown of the collagen in the skin and leading to stretch marks. These marks mostly appear on the abdomen and breasts, but they can also be seen on the thighs, buttocks, and upper arms. They can be darker or lighter than your skin tone or also appear reddish to purplish in colour. No cream, lotion, or ointment can get rid of stretch marks completely; however, they may fade a bit after pregnancy. Some actually can get darker after delivery also (see figure 6).

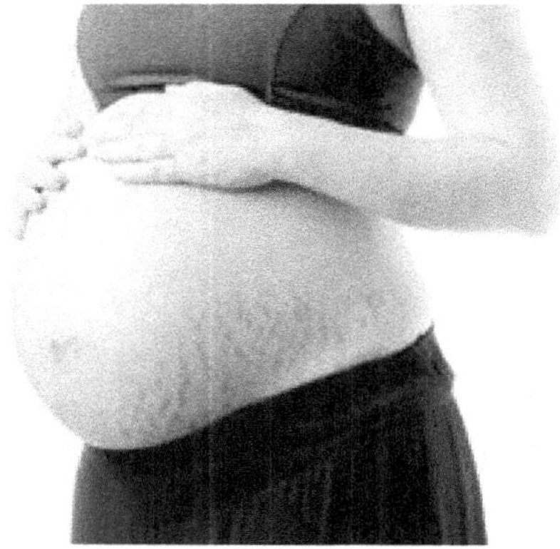

Figure 6. Stretch marks

Racing Heart: You may become very aware of your heart beating and may sometimes feel it racing. The heart rate increases in pregnancy to increase the amount of blood pumped towards the placenta. When other symptoms, such as chest pain or shortness of breath, occur with it, medical attention should be sought.

Nosebleed: Some women may have bleeding from the nose at this time. Do not become afraid; nosebleeds are common due to an increase in blood supply to the nose in pregnancy. Pinching the nose to apply pressure to the bleeding areas and holding the head back is helpful in halting the bleeding.

Heartburn: It is very common during pregnancy for women to experience a burning in the chest (sometimes associated with mild discomfort) or an unpleasant taste in the mouth. This is called acid reflux. If you are diagnosed with acid reflux prior to pregnancy it may worsen during pregnancy. These symptoms can be relieved with the use of antacids and other medications that decrease acid production in the stomach. Also consider position changes such as sleeping in the semi-recumbent position and avoiding foods like grapefruit, oranges, tomatoes and carbonated drinks. If you have symptoms of heartburn discuss it with your healthcare provider.

<u>SECOND TRIMESTER CHECKLIST</u>

- ✓ Decide if you will find out the sex of your baby.
- ✓ Ensure financial planning is in place.
- ✓ Begin to prepare other members of your household for your baby (including children and pets).
- ✓ Make time to spend with your spouse.
- ✓ Inform loved ones about your pregnancy.
- ✓ Start shopping for maternity clothes.

"Stand still and consider the wondrous works of God."

—Job 37:14 (KJV)

C H A P T E R   3

———— ⌁ ————

THE THIRD TRIMESTER

AFTER A LONG (but exciting) 28 weeks, we know you must be elated as time is drawing near when you will get to meet your baby. The suspense of it all will soon be over.

WEEKS 29–32

Your baby is now growing rapidly and gaining about half a pound per week. Fat begins to deposit underneath the skin, which adds to the baby's weight and aids in protection of the muscles, bones, and other internal organs. The baby's hair on the head also grows and thickens. Some babies, however, are not born with much hair. By this time your baby weights about 3.5 to 4 pounds and is about eighteen inches long.

WEEKS 33–37

Growth continues rapidly. The lungs are fully mature by 35 weeks, and the baby is able to breathe on its own outside the womb without assistance. However, a small percentage of babies born between 33 and 36 weeks may still require assistance breathing initially when born.

Your baby now weighs about 4.5 to 5.5 pounds and can reach six pounds by 37 weeks. Space in the amniotic sac is becoming very limited, and you will continue to feel movements. Your baby is ready to exit very soon!

<u>WEEKS 38–42</u>

You made it! You are now term! The baby is now ready to be born and can come at any time. Ninety-five percent of babies are born within two weeks of 40 weeks of pregnancy (that is, their due date time), and only 5 percent of women will in fact deliver exactly on their due date. While you wait, your baby is still growing in weight (but not in length.) The length of your baby is now about twenty-one inches, and the weight is about six to nine pounds. Your baby has also now turned into the position for delivery.

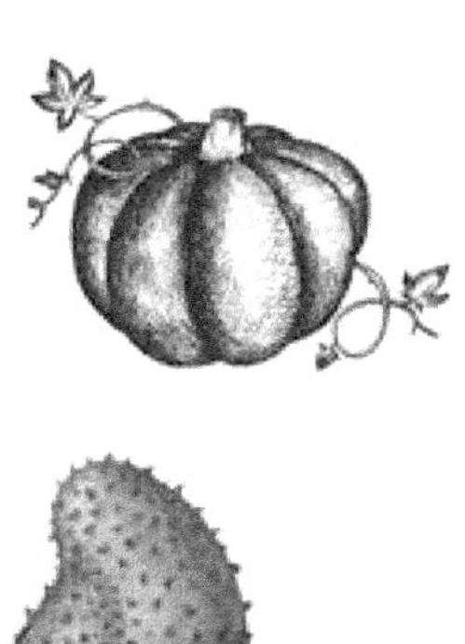

Figure 7. 29 weeks, Acorn Squash

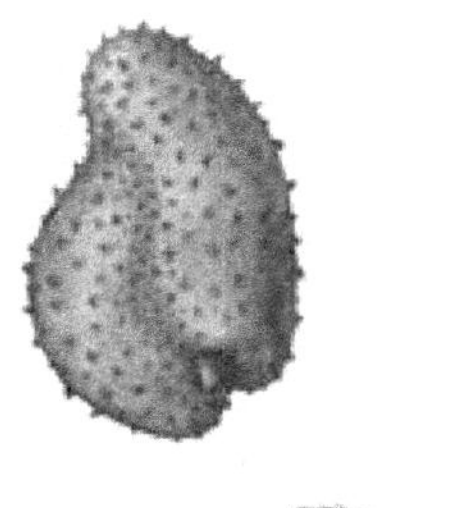

Figure 7A. 30 weeks, Soursop

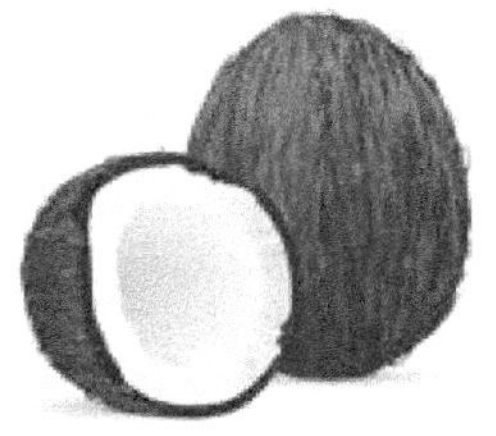

Figure 7B. 31 weeks, Coconut

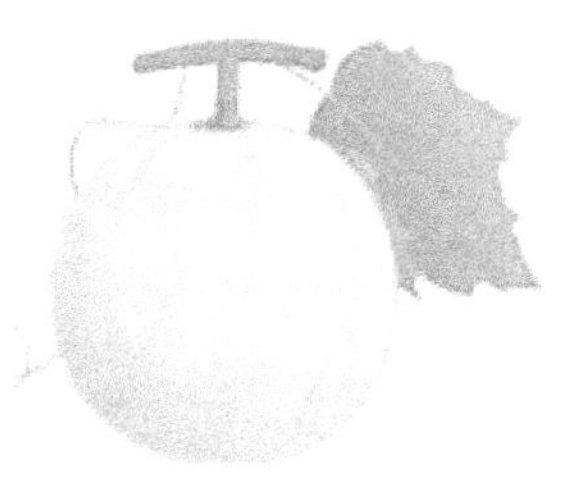

Figure 7C. 32 weeks, Honeydew Melon

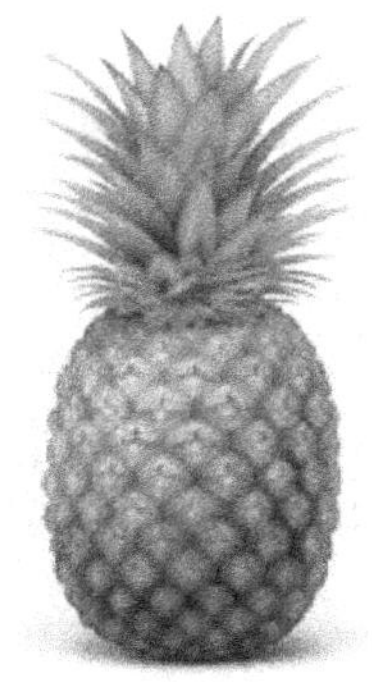

Figure 7D. 33 weeks, Pineapple

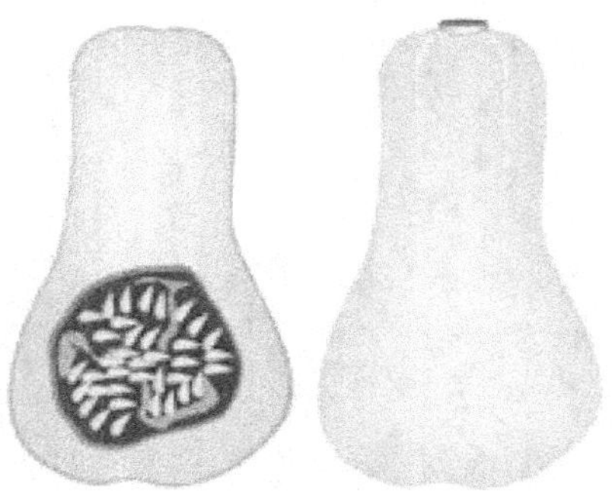

Figure 7E. 34 weeks, Butternut Squash

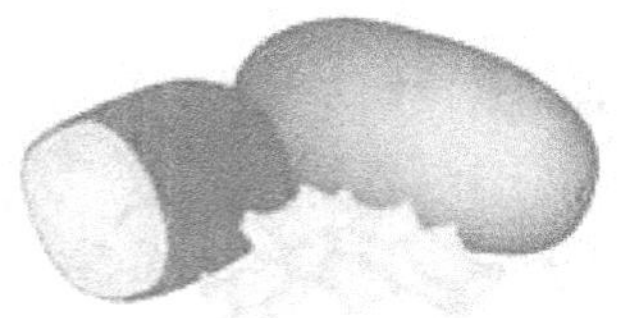

Figure 7F. 35 weeks, Winter Melon

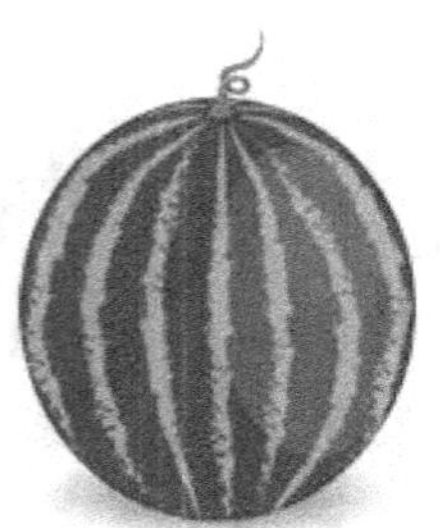

Figure 7G. 36 to 40 weeks, Watermelon

THIRD TRIMESTER TESTING

Ultrasound: In this trimester an ultrasound may be done for a variety of reasons, including assessing proper growth of the baby, estimating the fetal weight, and determining the position and lie of the baby (we will talk about this below).

POSITIONING OF THE BABY

During the middle of the third trimester, the fetus assumes its position (turns) to make its exit out into the world. This means a part of the fetus must be close to the neck of the womb and the bones of the pelvis through which it must pass. This is called *presentation*. Some women tend to be quite surprised when they attend a visit with their doctor or midwife and find out that the baby has already turned, as some expect to feel it occurring. Turning occurs during a series of movements over time, which is noted just to be normal fetal movements. There are several presentations that can occur:

Cephalic: Most babies will turn to be head down and the feet and buttock will be at the top of the womb (the *fundus*). The top of the head (known as the *vertex*) is what is often turned down (see figure 8). In a small number of women, however, the face or the ridge just above the eyes comes down first. Your doctor will determine on examination during labour if the baby will be able to be delivered safely in these latter two presentations; if not, a caesarean section would be required.

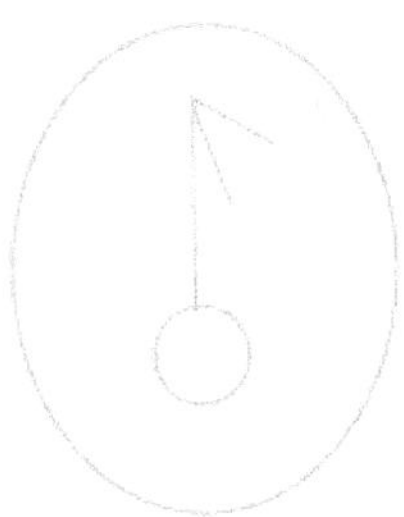

Figure 8.

Breech: This means that your baby is in a bottom-down position. Therefore, it exits the pelvis with its buttocks and legs as opposed to its head. If your baby is breech, you may feel discomfort under your ribs and become breathless as your baby's head presses up under your diaphragm. You may also feel some sharp kicks to your bladder. Breech presentation occurs in only about 3–5 percent of all pregnant women and is typically one of the following types:

- *Frank:* This is when the baby's buttock is entering the pelvis and both legs are extending up towards its head. Placing the baby in a somewhat "U" shape with the buttock being the curve of the "U" (see figure 8C).
- *Flexed:* With this type of breech the buttocks again are entering the pelvis but the legs are both bent at the knee, placing the baby in a position where the feet are bent up against the baby's tummy (see figure 8B).
- *Footling:* This is when one or both of the feet are hanging towards the pelvis. It is like the baby is standing on both feet or balancing on one leg (see figure 8A).

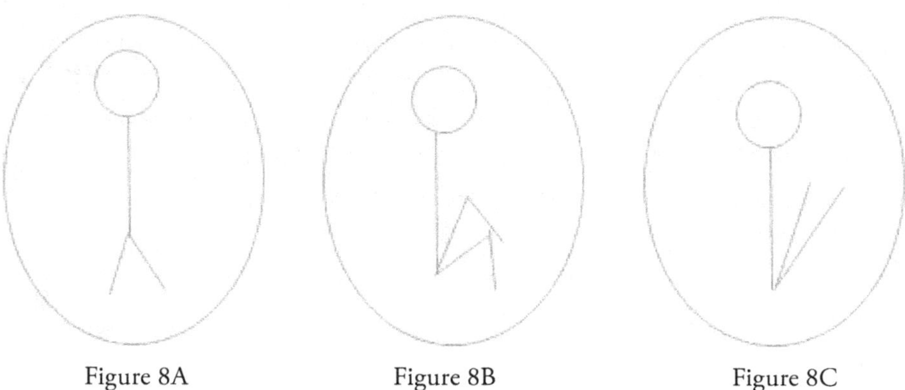

Figure 8A   Figure 8B   Figure 8C

What if my baby is breech near the end of my pregnancy?
Most babies would have turned head down by about 36 weeks gestation. For the babies that adopt a breech position, there are mainly two options available for approaching such a situation. Firstly, the baby may be able to be turned manually into the head down position by your physician. This is called *external*

cephalic version. Not all women are able to undergo this procedure. If you are pregnant with more than one baby, the placenta is in an abnormal position over the cervix, the baby is too large, or there is an abnormality in the uterus or with the baby are a few reasons why turning the baby may not be possible. The procedure is usually done in a hospital setting with the use of ultrasound and medications given to prevent contractions. You will also be placed on a monitor to ensure the baby's heart rate is normal during the procedure. Some women have no discomfort during the procedure; for others it can be painful. The chances of complications during the procedure are very low, but bleeding, a tear in the uterus, or the placenta separating from the uterine wall can occur.

Lie: A baby can only be delivered through the vagina if it is in longitudinal lie.

Longitudinal lie: This means the baby is lying straight (in an up/down position) (see figure 9A).

Transverse lie: This means that your baby is lying sideways (see figure 9B).

Oblique lie: This means your baby is lying at a slant in the womb (see figure 9C).

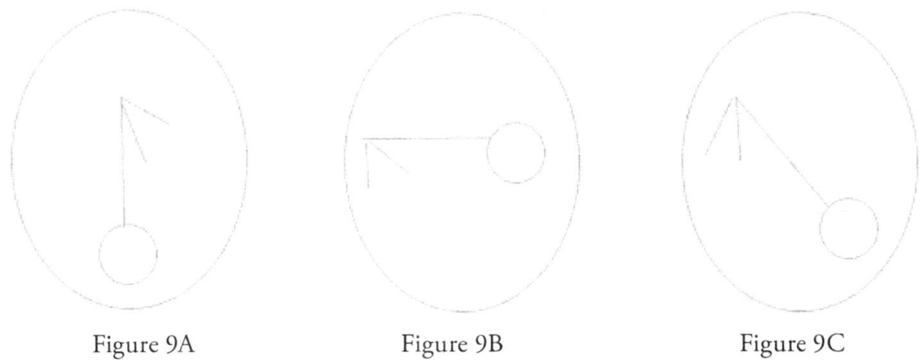

Figure 9A   Figure 9B   Figure 9C

BODY CHANGES AND OTHER EXPECTATIONS DURING THE THIRD TRIMESTER

Travel: Long airline or ship travel during this time can be risky in the event labour or complications occur. In the Bahamas, local airlines and boats will allow you to travel up until term. If you're intending to travel from a family island or to the mainland in whichever country you live in order to continue your antenatal care, it is best to travel before the third trimester. This decision can be made in corroboration with your healthcare provider.

Work: Some women find it increasingly difficult to work in the third trimester, while others are able to work up to term. It is important to discuss with your employer when you will commence maternity leave and plans for work postpartum.

Sex: Some may have an increase in the intensity of orgasms, and some women become disinterested in sex during this trimester, mainly because of all the changes occurring in the body. It may even be uncomfortable for some mothers. You can find other intimate acts (e.g., oral sex) to perform if intercourse is uncomfortable. As a couple, once you agree, then it is fine to have sexual intercourse up until you give birth. Orgasms in the late third trimester may cause leaking of milk from the breast in some women.

Fetal Movements: Your baby's movements during this time may not be as pronounced as weeks before. This is mainly because there is less space for the baby to move within your uterus. Now is the time to give the baby an eviction notice. You can keep a record of your baby's movement using a kick-count test. In this test you should monitor to see how long it takes you to feel ten movements. If it takes longer than two hours to feel this number of movements, contact your healthcare provider. Remember that your baby can sleep for periods of twenty to forty minutes and will not be moving during that time. Also, babies tend to be more active after you have had a meal.

COMMON COMPLAINTS

All the common complaints of the second trimester may continue into the third trimester or first begin in this trimester. Some additional issues you may encounter include:

Pelvic Pressure and Discomfort: As the baby's head moves downward into the pelvis, you may begin to experience more pelvic discomfort and pressure in the groin region and the hips. Sometimes there may be pelvic pain; if this happens it is best to sit down and rest awhile to relieve the pressure in the pelvis. It may be hard to find a comfortable position in the third trimester. Getting up, lying down, and walking around can all be a bit of a struggle. Here's the encouraging part of it all: you are almost at the end of your pregnancy journey.

Varicose Veins: These may be present on the legs and on the vulva. This is due to accumulation of blood in the veins that have been partly blocked by the expanding uterus. Some women find them painful or uncomfortable. Helpful tips include using support hosiery, elevating the legs, and side-sleeping.

Breathlessness: This a common symptom occurring in many pregnant women and most commonly in the third trimester. It may be present when resting or walking. It is most likely due to pregnancy-related changes, but there are diseases that affect the lungs that have to be taken into consideration also.

Frequent Urination: As your baby is growing, it places pressure on your bladder and you will likely find yourself making sure you always know where the nearest bathroom is.

Bloody Show: In the late third trimester (usually from about 37 weeks), you may notice passage of blood alone or mixed with a slimy, thick vaginal discharge. The spotting of blood can be pink or red. This means that your body is getting ready for your little one to make his or her entrance. It heralds the start of labour or may occur days to a few weeks before labour begins. If bleeding is heavy, you should contact your healthcare provider.

<u>THIRD TRIMESTER CHECKLIST:</u>

- ✓ Take a Lamaze class and/or lactation classes.
- ✓ Install your baby car seat and set up baby furniture towards the end of the third trimester.
- ✓ Take a visit to the place where you are going to give birth (if you have not already done so).
- ✓ Formulate a birth plan. Depending on the place of birth, this options may not be as flexible as you would like. Check with the hospital or birthing centre to see how feasible your proposed birth plan is.
- ✓ Choose your paediatrician. Depending on where you live, there are also community clinics provided by the government that provide free care for your baby after delivery.
- ✓ Consider having the house cleaned and baby-ready.
- ✓ Stock up on nonperishable food items.
- ✓ Pack your bag to take to the hospital. Below are some suggested items you should pack for you and your baby. (Mark the box if you have them ready!)

For Mother:

☐ *3 nightgowns/pajamas*	☐ *1 towel set*
☐ *1 robe*	☐ *1 comb and brush set*
☐ *6 panties*	☐ *1 tube of toothpaste*
☐ *2 good support bras*	☐ *1 toothbrush*
☐ *1 large pack of "overnight/ super" menstrual pads*	☐ *1 bottle of mouthwash*
	☐ *1 deodorant*
☐ *1 or 2 sets of bed linens (optional)*	☐ *1 light blanket*
	☐ *1 roll toilet tissue (optional)*

For Baby:

- ☐ *12 diapers*
- ☐ *2 small receiving blankets*
- ☐ *1 large receiving blanket*
- ☐ *1 burp cloth*
- ☐ *1 hypoallergenic bath set (lotion, wash, shampoo)*
- ☐ *1 hooded bath towel*
- ☐ *1 washcloth*
- ☐ *3 pairs of socks*
- ☐ *3 undershirts*

- ☐ *1 small pack of wipes*
- ☐ *3 nightgowns*
- ☐ *3 all-in-one sleepers or rompers*
- ☐ *2 caps for the baby's head*
- ☐ *1 comb and brush set*
- ☐ *1 "take home" outfit (optional)*

If you have gone through this checklist, you are ready for your bundle of joy. Labour can occur at any time, so be ready, just like we are admonished to be ready for Christ's return.

"Watch therefore, for you know neither the day nor the hour."

—Matthew 25:13 (ESV)

SECTION 2
LABOUR, DELIVERY, AND POSTPARTUM

"Shall I bring to the time of birth, and not cause delivery?" says the LORD.

—Isaiah 66:9 (NKJV)

C H A P T E R   4

INTRAPARTUM

INTRAPARTUM REFERS TO that period from the time a woman goes into labour up until the baby is born. This period can be very emotionally and physically taxing for the mother. The body is going through many changes that can sometimes bring out a myriad of emotions in the mother; some may even be volatile. It is important that mothers have good support during labour, as it helps in coping. In most hospitals and birthing centres, family members or friends are allowed in the birthing room.

PREPARING FOR LABOUR

There are many exciting ways that you and the father can prepare for the birth of your baby. You can take a birthing Lamaze class, which encourages you to use various techniques to deal with the pain and emotional changes that occur during labour. Many people will probably be giving you advice on how to prepare for labour; this advice may be quite beneficial, but it can also get you anxious and nervous about what will actually happen. It is important to go into the labour process with a clear mind. It is an exciting time; you want to focus all your energy on the life that you are about to usher into the world, without being overly anxious. Ask God to keep you calm.

"Do not be anxious about anything, but in every situation,
by prayer and petition, with thanksgiving, present your requests
to God."

—PHILIPPIANS 4:6 (NIV)

Another way to prepare for labour is to familiarize yourself with the stages of labour; continue reading this book and you will know just what to expect. Discuss your birth plan with your provider (e.g., if you wish not to receive pain relief during labour). Hospitals or birthing centres may allow you to tour the labour floor in preparation for delivery. If allowed you may wish to have dimed lights during labour or listen to your favorite calming music or Bible scriptures. It is important to discuss these things with your healthcare provider before the day of delivery.

LABOUR

Labour may begin as repeated uterine contractions associated with the thinning of the cervix (*effacement*) and the opening of the cervix (*dilation*). These uterine contractions can begin as cramps in the lower part of the abdomen (similar to period cramps) and progressively become more intense with a painful tightening and relaxing sensation of the abdomen.

The length of time spent in labour can vary from pregnancy to pregnancy and person to person. First-time mothers tend to labour longer than women who have delivered a baby before.

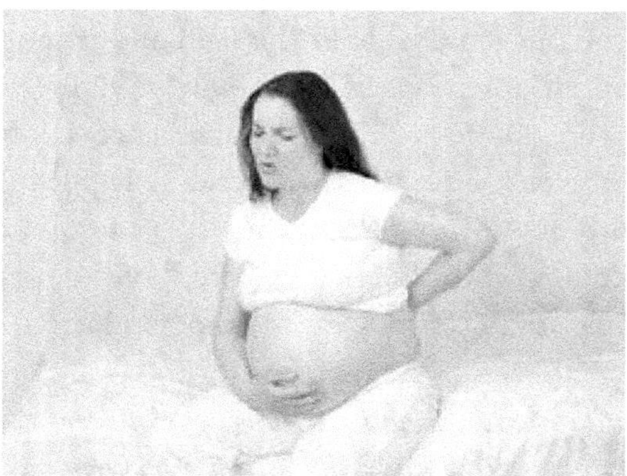

Figure 10. Labour pains, in the abdomen and back.

Labour and delivery is divided into three stages:

STAGE 1: EARLY (LATENT) AND ESTABLISHED (ACTIVE) LABOUR

In early labour the cervix dilates slowly but thins out. In the established phase of labour, dilation of the cervix occurs more quickly and effacement continues. For women in their first pregnancy, latent labour can last for up to eighteen hours, but for most women it averages at six to ten hours. During this time, having a good labour support, pain relief, and staying hydrated are important. Clear drinks, teas, and broths are best to consume during this time. Women in this phase can walk around and find other ways to cope with the pain. Contractions typically occur every ten to fifteen minutes during this time, lasting forty to ninety seconds. As the contractions become more frequent and intense, the active phase eventually begins.

How do I know when to go to the hospital?
Many women can remain at home during the latent phase of labour. It is important, however, when labour pains begin to call your healthcare provider to obtain advice as to what you should do. Contractions should be timed while at home. It is often difficult to know precisely when active labour begins, but as a general rule, once pains begin to intensify and become more frequent you should go to the hospital. Also, if your water breaks (even if there is no pain) or if you are bleeding, proceed to the hospital.

Once the cervix is about 4 cm dilated with frequent contractions, labour is established. The contractions now occur three to four times in a ten-minute period lasting about forty-five seconds each. During active labour, you will not be allowed to eat (or drink in some labour suites) in the event surgery is required.

Once you arrive at the hospital, several things will occur:

1. You will be examined to determine if you are indeed in labour. Once labour is diagnosed, you will be admitted formally to the labour and delivery unit.
2. Vitals will be taken, blood will be drawn to test your haemoglobin and reserve blood for transfusion (if needed), and an intravenous access will be placed in your arm. You may be required to sign forms

consenting to treatment and procedures during labour and caesarean section (if needed).

3. You will be asked to change your clothes, be given a gown to wear, and be placed on a labour bed (a bed with stirrups for your legs when it is time to push).

4. Some delivery units routinely give fleet enemas; however, this is not a requirement for labour.

5. Intravenous fluids will be started.

How does my healthcare provider know how I am progressing in labour?
During labour you will be examined every few hours. Two fingers of a gloved hand are placed in the vagina to determine how labour is progressing. The cervix undergoes changes in order to facilitate the baby's passage through the birth canal. The vagina is mostly a muscular organ that is able to stretch to accommodate the baby.

Dilation: At 10 cm dilated, the cervix is opened wide enough to accommodate the baby's head and body, and you are ready to push. For an easier understanding, 1 cm is about the diameter of a blueberry and 10 cm is the diameter of a regular bagel.

Effacement: When the cervix is fully effaced (100 percent effaced), it can feel almost paper-thin.

Station: This is how close the widest part of the baby's head is to two bony triangular projections on the mother's pelvis called the *ischial spines*. It determines how the baby's head is descending downward towards the pelvic inlet for delivery. Station is measured in centimetres away from the ischial spines. The type of pelvis that best accommodates the head is called the gynaecoid pelvis.

Contractions: These are monitored by a midwife or nurse feeling your abdomen with her hand about every thirty minutes. This gives subjective information on the intensity and frequency of your contractions. These are also recorded on a cardiotocogram.

Cardiotocogram (CTG): This records a tracing of the baby's heart rate and your contractions during labour on a special type of paper. This allows your

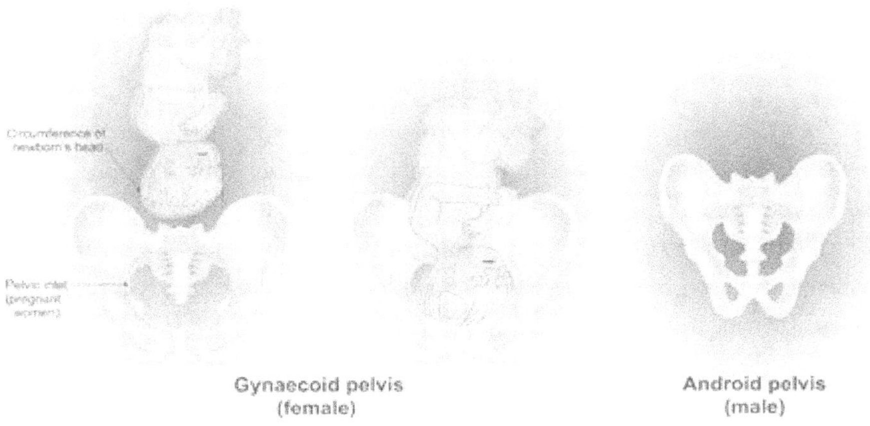

Figure 11. Fetal Station and Pelvis Types

provider to know how well the baby is tolerating labour. In order to obtain this tracing, two probes leading from the CTG machine are attached to your abdomen. If the tracing is poor, which can be due to several factors, a sterile probe may need to be attached to the skin of the baby's head through the vagina, and this is called a *fetal scalp probe.*

What if I am not progressing in labour?
If cervical dilatation and effacement are slow you may be given additional fluids via the veins, or your amniotic sac may need to be artificially ruptured. This procedure is quick (about one minute or less) and done by inserting a small instrument into the vagina that punctures the sac. If your contractions are infrequent or irregular, a medication that is the man-made form of oxytocin (Pitocin® or Syntocinon®) may be given to you continuously through the veins. This will cause your contractions to come closer together and get stronger. This aims to cause further dilatation and effacement of the cervix.

How does my baby move to get out of my uterus during labour?
During labour your baby goes through a series of movements and turns in order to move downward and through the pelvis and vaginal canal for exit

out of the vagina. The position of your baby can be determined by vaginal examinations during labour.

What about the pain, will something be given for that?
You will have the options for pain relief in labour or there may be none at all. Some women are able to tolerate high levels of pain with minimal discomfort. However, if you are unable to cope with the pain, you should inform your healthcare provider. Several options are available for pain relief and these are discussed further in this chapter.

Stage 2: Delivery of the Baby

When your cervix is 10 cm dilated and fully thinned out, it is time to push. You have been waiting for this moment for so long, so now is your time to shine and put in a lot of effort. When this stage arrives, women often have an urge to push. If you have regional anaesthesia (discussed in chapter 4), you may not feel this urge, but don't worry, your healthcare provider will let you know when it is time to push. Pushing for labour is bearing down as if you are trying to pass faeces. With each push the baby comes further downward. You should only push during a contraction and rest in between. It is important to follow your provider's instructions on pushing, and they will advise you when to push forcefully or to give small pushes and when to stop pushing. As the head is being delivered, you may feel an intense burning sensation in the vagina as the tissues are stretched. Some women need an intentional cut made in the vagina to allow room for delivery of the head called an *episiotomy*. There is some relief of pain when the head is delivered, until the shoulders and then the body is delivered. The baby is out! You are filled with happiness and joy at the site of your baby. God truly is awesome in taking you success-fully through this journey. Once your baby is deemed well and the cord is cut, he or she may be placed on your chest to allow you to bond with your baby. The father of your baby, or even another loved one whom you choose, may be allowed to cut the cord. If you would like that, you should discuss it in your birth plan with your healthcare provider in the third trimester of pregnancy. Finally, if you got an episiotomy, it will be stitched (sutured) after the third stage of labour is complete.

What if I have been pushing for a while and the baby still does not come?
There can be several reasons why this stage can be prolonged. If your baby is very large, your pelvis is considered small (*cephalopelvic disproportion*), or if the baby's head is in an abnormal position, it may make pushing difficult. Your healthcare provider will examine you to assess what the cause may be. Sometimes you may become extremely tired after pushing for a long time, or the abnormal position of the head may need to be corrected with a method called *operative vaginal delivery*. This entails using a vacuum cup or forceps to assist in getting the baby's head out of the birth canal. In some instances, the best option when this stage is prolonged is to proceed to a caesarean section. However, you and your healthcare provider will determine the best plan of action to ensure the best outcome for you and your baby.

Stage 3: Delivery of the Placenta

Now that the baby is out, most of your work is done. However, your healthcare provider still has to remove the placenta. This usually occurs within the next five to thirty minutes. Upon its delivery, the placenta is inspected to make sure none of it is left behind.

If the placenta has not separated and delivered within thirty minutes, it may need to be manually removed. In this procedure you will be given a medication for pain, and one hand of your provider is inserted into the vagina and then the uterus to remove the placenta. Even with pain medication this procedure may be a bit uncomfortable. If the placenta is unable to be removed on the labour floor, you will be taken to the operating theatre and given anaesthesia that allows for better removal of the placenta.

OPERATIVE VAGINAL DELIVERY

Once pushing begins in the second stage of labour, it takes about one to two hours for the baby to be delivered. Some women who are first-time moms and have a particular type of pain medication (regional anaesthesia) may be allowed to push for up to three hours. However, most persons that have reached the two-hour mark and the head has not delivered will likely not deliver the head on their own efforts. This is where operative vaginal delivery comes into play. These are measures used to assist in the delivery of the fetal head (which is sitting in the vagina and very close to coming out) and can include devices such as a vacuum cup (*ventouse delivery*) or forceps.

In a ventouse delivery, a small cup (usually made of plastic, but in some delivery units it is metal) is placed on the baby's head and suction is applied to keep the cup attached. As you push with a contraction, traction is placed on the cup to lift the head out of the vagina. When a vacuum is used, a small swelling will be noticed on the baby's head where the cup was applied, which is not harmful or painful and will go down in several days to weeks. Forceps delivery uses a metal instrument that has two parts that are inserted into the vagina on of either side of the baby's face and head. Again, with a contraction and pushing, the head is lifted out of the vagina. These methods can be very helpful, particularly when you have been pushing for a long time and are fatigued or if the baby is in distress and needs to be delivered right away. You and your doctor will determine if a caesarean section or an operative vaginal delivery is a better option for you at this point.

Operative vaginal delivery, even when done correctly and is successful, can have complications that include cuts on the baby's head or face, bleeding just below the scalp, and bleeding within the baby's brain. These complications are infrequent, however.

SHOULDER DYSTOCIA

Shoulder dystocia is when there is difficulty in delivering the baby's shoulders after the head has been delivered. This is an emergency and will require quick manoeuvres in order to prevent lack of oxygen to the baby.

When a shoulder dystocia is occurring, there may be many healthcare personnel in the room and they will be instructing you. It can be very overwhelming, but know that all of the apparent chaos is actually quite organized in an effort to deliver your baby. Someone may lift your legs higher towards your chest, and someone else may be pressing on your *mons* (the triangular region that is below your bikini line area), while your healthcare provider continues to deliver the baby. Once delivered, the baby is passed onto the paediatrician for assessment. Some babies unfortunately suffer nerve damage that affects the movement of the arm (this resolves in 90 percent of infants by one year of age). Others complications of shoulder dystocia to the baby include a broken arm or clavicle. An episiotomy may need to be done in order to make room for delivering the shoulders. Some infants that are unable to be delivered within five minutes may have neurological impairment or may even die. Shoulder dystocia is an unpredictable event but may occur with larger babies.

ANAESTHESIA AND ANALGESIC OPTIONS FOR LABOUR AND DELIVERY

> *"When a woman is giving birth, she has sorrow because her hour has come, but when she has delivered the baby, she no longer remembers the anguish, for joy that a human being has been born into the world."*

> —JOHN 16:21 (ESV)

When it comes to using anaesthesia in childbirth, most women fall into one of three categories:

1. Those who are quite certain they will want pain relief.
2. Those who are unsure of their pain relief options and how they will affect their labour and delivery.
3. Those who would prefer to give birth without any pain relief.

No matter which category you think you will fall into, it is important for you to know how anaesthesia and pain relief are used in labour and delivery as the category you fall into may change.

Obstetrical anaesthesia is different from any other type of anaesthesia in that there are two patients involved—you and your baby. Labour is unpredictable. It can range anywhere from relatively quick and easy to painful and exhausting. An important point to remember is that everyone experiences pain differently. Only you will know the level of pain you're experiencing, so you should never feel bad about asking for pain relief. Pregnant women, in fact, are expected to experience some level of pain based on the Word of God:

> *"Then He said to the woman, 'I will sharpen the pain of your pregnancy, and in pain you will give birth.'"*

> —Genesis 3:16 (NLT)

Pain during labour is caused by different actions that may be happening in the body. For example, uterine muscle contractions as well as pressure on the cervix, bladder, and bowels may be sources of pain. Pain may also happen from the stretching of the birth canal and vagina when the baby is being delivered. The way a contraction feels may be different for each woman and from one pregnancy to the next. Labour contractions may cause extreme pain or a dull ache in your back and lower abdomen, along with pressure in the pelvis. Some women might also feel pain in their sides and thighs.

It is important for you to learn what pain relief options are available during childbirth. Your healthcare provider will most likely talk about your pain options before you go into labour. Getting pain relief is important as agreed on by the American Congress of Obstetricians and Gynecologists and the Royal College of Obstetricians and Gynaecologists.

Remember, however, that your pain relief choices might be governed by certain circumstances of your labour and delivery. Throughout your labour, your healthcare provider will assess your progress and comfort to help you choose a pain relief technique. Pain relief may affect your view of the overall labour experience.

Your healthcare provider might ask an anaesthesiologist (a doctor who specializes in pain relief) to talk with you about pain relief during labour and answer your questions. Anaesthetics block all pain and sensation, whereas analgesics only lessen the pain. There are several different forms of anaesthesia administered for childbirth. They may be used independently or in conjunction with one another. Some of the most commonly administered anaesthetics include the following:

LOCAL ANAESTHESIA

This is a series of local injections can make you more comfortable for delivery and for the placement of sutures, if you need them. Local anaesthetic to numb your vaginal area in preparation for delivery is called a *pudendal block*.

REGIONAL ANAESTHESIA

Also called *epidural, spinal,* or *systemic anaesthesia*, regional anaesthesia is the most common and effective pain relief. Regional anaesthesia greatly reduces or eliminates pain throughout the birthing process. It can also be used if a caesarean birth becomes necessary. An anaesthesiologist administers it during labour to reduce discomfort, and with each type, medicines are placed near the nerves in your lower back to block pain in a wide region of your body while you stay awake.

- *Epidural:* A local anaesthetic delivered through a small catheter placed in the small of the back, just outside the spinal canal. Medicine is given through the catheter when needed. The tube is left in place during the labour course. If a caesarean section is needed, a stronger dose of medicine can be given through the tube. A benefit of the epidural is that it allows most women to fully participate in the birth experience (to continue to feel touch and pressure) while relieving most, if not all, of the pains of labour. In most cases the anaesthesiologist will start the epidural once labour is established. But, in some cases, it may be desirable to place the epidural earlier.
- *Spinal:* This anaesthetic is similar to an epidural, but it is administered with a small needle into the spinal canal in the form of single injection. Although a small amount of medication is required, its

effects are felt much faster. You may feel numb and need assistance in moving during the delivery. Spinal anaesthetics are sometimes used for delivery by caesarean section or when forceps use is indicated.

- *Combined Spinal-Epidural or CSE:* This is a combination of the above two. The initial spinal injection makes you numb quickly but can also be used to give more anaesthetic if needed.

How is regional anaesthesia given?
Your anaesthesiologist will inject medicines near the nerves in your lower back to block the discomfort of contractions. The medicine will be injected while you are either sitting up or lying on your side.

After reviewing your medical history and asking you some questions, your anaesthesiologist will numb an area on your lower back with a local anaesthetic. A special needle is inserted into this numb area to find the exact location to inject the anaesthetic medicine. After putting in the medicine, your anaesthesiologist removes the needle. A tiny plastic tube called an epidural catheter may be left in place after the needle is removed to deliver medicines as needed throughout labour.

When is regional anaesthesia given?
The best time to administer regional anaesthesia may differ depending on you and your baby's response to labour. If you request regional anaesthesia, your healthcare provider will contact your anaesthesiologist and together they will discuss with you the risks, benefits, and timing of regional anaesthesia.

If you request regional anaesthesia, you might receive epidural or spinal anaesthesia, or a combination of the two. Your healthcare provider will select the type of regional anaesthesia based on your general health and the progress of your labour.

Will a regional block affect my baby?
Considerable research has shown that regional anaesthesia is safe for you and your baby.

How soon does regional anaesthesia take effect and how long does it last?
Epidural anaesthesia starts working within ten to twenty minutes after the medicine has been injected. Pain relief from epidural anaesthesia lasts as long as your labour, since more medicine can always be given through the catheter.

Spinal anaesthesia starts working immediately after the medicine has been injected. Pain relief lasts about two and one half hours.

How numb will regional anaesthesia make me feel?
Although you will feel significant pain relief, you might still be aware of mild pressure from your contractions. You might also feel pressure when your healthcare provider examines you.

Do I have to stay in bed after regional anaesthesia?
If you have received a combined spinal and epidural, your anaesthesiologist can tailor the anaesthesia to allow you to sit in a lounge chair or walk. Walking or sitting might even help your progress in labour. If you are interested, ask your anaesthesiologist about a "walking epidural." But, keep in mind this depends on the policy of your hospital and availability of this type of anaesthesia.

Will a regional block slow my labour?
In some women, contractions might slow after regional anaesthesia for a short period of time. Most women find that regional anaesthesia helps them to relax and actually improves their contraction pattern while allowing them to rest.

If I have regional anaesthesia, will I be able to push?
Yes. Regional anaesthesia allows you to rest comfortably while your cervix dilates. When your cervix is completely dilated and it is time to push, you will have energy in reserve. Regional anaesthesia may affect your ability to feel the contractions but should not affect your ultimate ability to push. Pushing may take a little longer, but the regional anaesthesia will make pushing more comfortable for you.

Are there any side effects of regional anaesthesia?
Your anaesthesiologist takes special precautions to prevent complications, such as reviewing your history and laboratories prior to the procedure, making sure you are well hydrated, and paying attention to your anatomy. Although complications are rare, some side effects might include:

- *Decreased blood pressure*: You will receive intravenous fluids, and your blood pressure will be carefully monitored and treated to prevent this from happening.
- *Mild itching during labour*: If itching becomes bothersome, your anaesthesiologist may recommend medication to treat it.
- *Headache*: Drinking fluids and taking pain tablets can help relieve headaches after regional anaesthesia. If the headache persists, tell your anaesthesiologist and other medicines can be ordered for you.
- *Local anaesthetic reaction*: While local anaesthetic reactions are rare, they can be serious. Be sure to tell your anaesthesiologist if you become dizzy or develop ringing in your ears.

Also be sure to listen and follow the instructions of the anaesthesiologist and your healthcare provider.

Sedation

Narcotics or tranquilizers are analgesics administered as an injection or intravenously and can help reduce the pain of labour but will not stop the pain entirely. They are also used to ease the anxiety that sometimes accompanies the delivery process. They may make you and your baby sleepy. They are mainly used during labour to help you relax if other methods are not available.

What Your Anaesthesiologist Should Know

In order for your anaesthesiologist to determine which type of anaesthesia is best for you and your baby, it is important that you inform your anaesthesiologist about:

- Food and drink intake for the last several hours, any allergies to medications, or medications that you have recently been taking.
- History of difficulty breathing after anaesthesia.
- History of lower back problems or surgeries.
- History of infections such as HIV.
- Any respiratory problems, such as asthma, bronchitis, or pneumonia, or if you have a cold, sore throat, or flu.
- Special medical concerns such as cardiac disease, diabetes, and asthma, among others.

If you are a woman with any of these conditions, it is especially important that you meet with an anaesthetist prior to going into labour so they can assess you before labour and develop a plan for your labour that will meet your needs and minimize your risk.

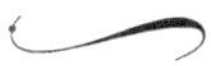

INDUCTION OF LABOUR

When labour has to be commenced artificially using a variety of methods and medications, this is called *induction of labour*. When labour starts on its own, it is called *spontaneous labour*. There are many reasons why a person may need to be induced instead of awaiting spontaneous labour. By far the most common reason is when the pregnancy has gone past the estimated date of delivery (*postdate*). Other reasons include postterm pregnancy (past 42 weeks gestation), if the baby is not growing well (*fetal growth restriction*), rhesus incompatibility, diabetes in pregnancy, infection within the amniotic sac (*chorioamnionitis*), if the baby has died within the womb (*stillbirth*), hypertension in pregnancy, sickle cell disease, or kidney disease.

When it has been decided that induction of labour is required in your pregnancy, you will be admitted to the labour unit of your hospital. The baby will be monitored during the induction process with a nonstress test. This test records a tracing of the baby's heart rate on paper and correlates with how well the baby is doing in the uterus during the induction of labour process. If there is any evidence that the baby is in distress (seen as changes of the heart rate on the tracing), emergent delivery may be required. A vaginal exam is done to assess the readiness of the cervix. As stated earlier, the cervix goes through changes of softening and dilating as labour progresses. If the cervix is not ready for labour, a process called *cervical ripening* is done.

Prostaglandins

Cervical ripening can be done using medications called *prostaglandins* (PG), which are placed in the vagina or given by mouth. Prostaglandins works in two ways; they ripen the cervix and also can stimulate contractions and therefore induce labour. Commonly used PGs include *dinoprostone* (as a vaginal gel or tablet) and *misoprostol* (as tablets, oral or vaginal).

Dilators

A vaginal insert containing *Laminaria japonica (which is a type of kelp)* is placed in the cervix and it absorbs fluid around it causing it to expand and stimulate changes in the cervix and contractions. Other methods that work by stretching and dilating the cervix are catheters—that is, inflating the balloon end of a catheter (known as a Foley's), inserting it into the cervix, and instilling a sterile fluid between the amniotic sac and the lower uterus.

Stripping the Membranes

Stripping (or sweeping) of the membranes is a method whereby your healthcare provider inserts two fingers into the vagina, then into an open cervix and attempts to separate the amniotic sac from the lower part of the uterus. This aims to stimulate the release of natural prostaglandins in the body that soften the cervix and stimulate contractions. Stripping of the membranes can be done starting the last two weeks prior to your due date (around 38 weeks gestation). Research on this method has shown that it may decrease the chance of you going past your due date and therefore requiring other methods of induction.

OXYTOCIN AND AMNIOTOMY

If your cervix is already ripe when examined, other methods of induction that can be used are administering a synthetic (man-made) form of oxytocin (which is similar to the natural hormone oxytocin produced by the brain and released into the body during spontaneous labour). Breaking the water sac (called *amniotomy*) is another method and is often not done alone but in conjunction with oxytocin administration.

Women who are induced sometimes describe the pain as being more than if labour had occurred on its own. However, pain medications can be administered if pain becomes intolerable for you.

Many traditional methods have been tried to induce labour too, including teas, sexual intercourse, castor oil, and nipple stimulation. Of these, nipple stimulation is the only one proven to cause uterine contractions; however, you should not try this method without consultation with your healthcare provider.

Although induction of labour is a safe and well-monitored procedure, complications can still occur with the use of some of the methods. These complications are:

- A decrease in the fetal heart rate
- Frequent (too numerous) contractions in a ten-minute period
- Infection
- Cord prolapse
- Uterine rupture (which is very rare)

Your healthcare provider will monitor you closely during the induction process to detect if any of these complications occur.

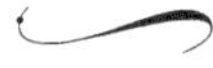

CAESAREAN SECTION

Caesarean sections (C-sections) have greatly lessened the number of women who have died or lost their babies in recent centuries due to pregnancy complications that made vaginal delivery a risk or that required urgent delivery. A caesarean section is delivery of the baby through an incision that is made on the abdomen and the uterus.

The course of your pregnancy can change from one moment to the next, and although the aim for most women is a vaginal delivery, your birth plan can be changed suddenly if a circumstance arises that requires caesarean section. It may be an *elective caesarean section* (in which a day that is suitable for the mother and the obstetrician is chosen) or it may be an *emergency caesarean section* in which the surgery is needed immediately partway through regular labour and delivery. Some conditions place you at greater chances of requiring a C-section than others, but there are many reasons why you may require one:

- C-section delivery in the past
- Problem with the baby's heart rate
- Cessation of dilation and effacement of the cervix
- Mass or fibroid blocking the birth canal
- Cephalopelvic disproportion
- An abnormality with the baby
- Large baby (*fetal macrosomia*)
- A very small or preterm baby
- Abnormal presentation or positioning of the baby
- Twins or more than two babies
- Problems with the placenta or umbilical cord
- Heavy vaginal bleeding
- Seizures due to pregnancy (*eclampsia*)
- Cancer of the cervix
- Present outbreak of genital warts or herpes near or at the time of delivery

It can be very scary for a mother who had all intentions to deliver vaginally to be told she requires a caesarean section. However, when you place your fear in the hands of Jesus, His "perfect love casts out fear," according to 1 John 4:18 (ESV).

A caesarean section is done in the operating theatre and most commonly under regional anaesthesia (which allows the mother to be awake during the procedure, but unable to feel any pain). This allows the mother and father (or whomever else is in the room) to experience the birth. Most operating theatres only allow one adult in with you for support. In some emergencies, however, you may have to be put to sleep for the procedure.

All persons in the room will be dressed in operating-room scrubs and sterile attire for the surgery. A paediatrician will be there to assess the baby after delivery. You will be attached to several monitors during the procedure. An incision of about 8 to 10 cm is made in a horizontal direction just at the bikini line (called a *Pfannenstiel incision*). Once the uterus is reached, an incision is made usually on its lower part (called a *transverse incision*). The baby and then the placenta are delivered through this incision. Afterward all the tissue layers are stitched closed with a suture material that dissolves over time (so you don't have to have stitches removed after a C-section). You will be transferred to an area where you will be monitored for a while (the recovery room also known as the *postanaesthetic care unit*) before returning to your room on the maternity floor.

A scripture that you can meditate on if you have been told that you require a caesarean section is Jeremiah 30:17 (NLT):

> *"'I will give you back your health and heal your wounds,' says the Lord."*

Although caesarean sections are a common surgery, they are still a major surgery and rarely complications can happen, including damage to your bladder or bowel structures, infection, blood clots, excessive blood loss, risk of losing your uterus if bleeding is uncontrollable, and lacerations to the baby, which are usually small and heal without problems. These above complications occur in less than 2 percent of all caesarean sections.

Recovery time from a caesarean section takes usually around six to eight weeks; however, once there are no major complications, you will be moving around (short distances) and even eating in as little as eight hours after your surgery, and you can usually be discharged from hospital by the third day after your procedure. Initially walking will be painful but will improve. You will be sent home with pain medications and antibiotics to decrease the risk of infection.

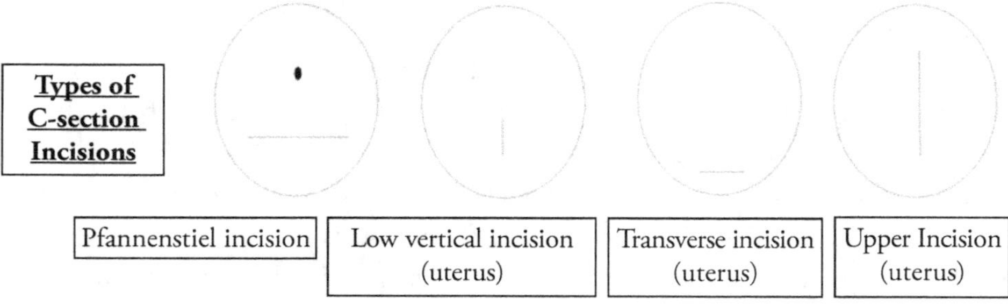

Figure 12. Types of C-section Incisions

TRIAL OF LABOUR AFTER CAESAREAN SECTION

Once a C-section, always a C-section? This is a question we are sure someone is wondering after having had a caesarean section. Well, the answer is: not necessarily. We will explain!

Trial of labour after caesarean section (TOLAC) is an attempt at vaginal delivery after a woman has had a caesarean section in the past. Your doctor may give you this option during the antenatal period. The alternative to TOLAC is having an elective repeat caesarean section.

In women who have not completed child bearing and wish to have more children, TOLAC may be an acceptable option. It has the advantages of a quick recovery after delivery, less blood lost, and less chance of infection when it is compared with having a repeat C-section. There is also the avoidance of major surgery and having multiple C-sections if you desire more children. The largest risk of TOLAC is a small chance of the tissues of the uterus tearing (in the area where the previous surgery was done), called *uterine rupture*. This happens in one in every two hundred (0.5 percent) women who undergo

TOLAC. Women are closely monitored in labour but should this happen, you would require an emergency caesarean section.

The more caesarean sections you have, the greater chance of having excessive blood loss at surgery or damage to organs that are close to the uterus, which includes the bladder, bowel, and two tubes that extend from the kidneys into the bladder (*ureters*). If the placenta is unable to be detached from the uterus after delivery of the fetus, this can lead to uncontrollable bleeding at surgery, the need for blood transfusions, and possibly the need for removal of the uterus in order to save your life. An advantage of choosing to have an elective repeat caesarean section is, if you have decided that you do not want any more children, your fallopian tubes can be tied at the same time of the surgery for convenience.

Some women, however, are not good candidates for TOLAC, especially if your last C-section was less than a year prior, if there has been previous surgery on the upper part of your uterus (including a classical caesarean section), you have had uterine rupture before, the baby is estimated to be very large, or there is another reason you are unable to give vaginal birth. You should have a thorough discussion with your physician, and together you both can decide which option is best for you, as every woman's circumstances are different.

C H A P T E R   5

POSTPARTUM CARE AND COMPLICATIONS

PHYSICAL CHANGES IN THE POSTPARTUM PERIOD

MANY CHANGES TAKE place in the postpartum period that support the new baby and return the mother's body to its state prior to pregnancy.

UTERUS

The uterus contracts intermittently after delivery in order to seal off blood vessels and decrease bleeding. These contractions aid in a process called *involution* in which the uterus is returning to its normal prepregnancy size. These contracts may be felt and can be painful. Immediately after delivery of the placenta, the uterus shrinks in size (due to the contractions) and can be felt just at the belly button as a hard, smooth structure (like a round golf ball, just a bit bigger).

LOCHIA

Lochia is the bloody discharge that comes from the lining of the uterus down through the vagina after delivery. It is initially red in colour and heavy (like a heavy period). Then, over the course of a few days to weeks, it becomes lighter, thinner, and pink in colour to eventually a clear discharge before stopping in about two to four weeks. This bleeding comes from the site within the uterus that the placenta was attached to. Over the course of days to weeks, the blood vessels in this area close off due to contractions of the uterus and bleeding decreases.

If you saturate your sanitary pad at home in an hour for two hours or more this is too much lochia and you should contact your healthcare provider (see the section on *postpartum haemorrhage* below). Also, if the lochia has a foul-smelling odour this may indicate an infection of the uterus (endometritis) and you should call your provider.

Passing Urine

If you have had a vaginal delivery, passing urine may be a bit difficult in the first few days after delivery. This is because as the baby passes through the birth canal it rests on your bladder and the opening of your bladder (called the *urethra*), which causes some swelling. It usually goes away in a few days. You may also notice leaking of urine as well, and this is because the delivery can make the bladder muscles a little weak in some women. This will usually go away, but if it does not contact your healthcare provider.

Passing Faeces

Initially passing faeces may be a bit painful, especially if you have had an episiotomy. Stool softeners may help in this situation. If you notice that faeces is coming through your vagina, this is not normal and you should contact your healthcare provider. This can happen if tears occurred during delivery and extended into the back passage causing an abnormal connection between the vagina and rectum.

Breastfeeding

The initial time spent with your baby is important; during this time you can bond and establish breastfeeding. As stated in an earlier chapter, the breasts begin to produce milk during pregnancy and it is after delivery that milk lets down due to stimulation by a chemical called *dopamine* released from nerve endings and a hormone from the pituitary gland called *prolactin*. The first milk is called *colostrum*, and it is thick, yellowish in colour (or may even be clear), and high in protein. It also contains antibodies that help your baby fight off infection.

Your baby should be placed on the breast to suckle frequently (though it may only be for short periods at a time in the first few days because the breasts are not full with milk as yet). The more the baby suckles the greater the milk supply. Colostrum is power-packed, containing so much goodness in small volumes at a time. In a few days "mature" milk comes down, and this is more cream to white in colour and contains more fats and sugars (carbohydrates) than colostrum.

AFTER A CAESAREAN SECTION

- Pain may still be present, albeit minimal, especially when walking around and even with prescribed medication, but this begins to decrease in the days after. Continue walking a little more each day. If the pain becomes unbearable, you should return to your healthcare provider.
- Rest when needed and do not participate in any exercising or strenuous activities or heavy lifting (except lifting the baby) for at least six weeks.
- You may feel a sudden pain at your incision site when coughing; holding a pillow over the site may help.
- You will be required to return a few days after your surgery to check on your wound to ensure that it is healing well.

AFTER A VAGINAL DELIVERY

- You will be seen in about two weeks to ensure that you are breastfeeding well and have no difficulty passing urine or faeces. Keep hydrated and eat fruits and vegetables to help avoid constipation. Haemorrhoids tend to improve slowly after delivery.
- If you had an episiotomy, you should sit in a warm bath with Epsom salt (magnesium sulphate) about three times a day for fifteen minutes each time for a week and this will promote healing and reduce pain. The area will be inspected to make sure it is not infected but is

healing well. Even if you haven't had an episiotomy, it is not uncommon to have vaginal pain; this will go away eventually. Persistent pain should be discussed with your healthcare provider.

When Can I Have Sex after Delivery?

Sex is an important part of a relationship and for various reasons women may have been unable to fully enjoy sex during pregnancy. So, you want get back to the fun (but be careful, that fun was what got you pregnant!) The Bible speaks about abstaining from sex for prayer purposes until the husband and wife mutually agree to come back together (1 Corinthians 7:5); the same should apply after having a baby. Make sure that you are healed and not experiencing any discomfort. It may or may not be uncomfortable the first time. Some women have decreased sexual drive initially, which can be due to the overall fatigue from the delivery or the demands associated with a new baby and your family. Even the way your body is viewed may have changed, and vaginal dryness causing painful intercourse can be a factor also. Vaginal dryness may be more common if you are breastfeeding, as the hormone that helps in milk production can cause dryness. Vaginal lubricants can be used during intercourse for this. Orgasms after delivery may cause leaking of milk from the breast in some women (who are still breastfeeding). Rarely, some women may feel guilty because in some first-time breastfeeding moms it may stimulate sexual arousal. However, as you get accustomed to breastfeeding, this should eventually stop occurring.

For most women intercourse can resume within four to six weeks after a caesarean section and within days to weeks after a vaginal delivery. It is best to wait until all heavy lochia has decreased. If you required an episiotomy, you should wait at least four weeks to ensure the site is healed and the stitches are not disrupted as a result of intercourse. Some nonbreastfeeding mothers can ovulate as early as twenty-eight days after delivery; however, the earliest for most women is forty-two days. A misconception that some women have is that they must see their period first before they ovulate. This is not true; you can ovulate and become pregnant without having a menstruation after birth. So, when resuming sexual intercourse, you should ensure that you are using a form of birth control, especially if you had a caesarean section. A pregnancy occurring prior to healing from a caesarean section can increase the chances of uterine rupture.

What About My Hair, Will It Return to "Normal"?

As the pregnancy hormones diminish you may find that your hair loss seems to increase as more of your hair follicles enter the "resting" phase as compared to your pregnancy. You will find that in six to twelve months your hair may return to prepregnancy status. In the interim, you may want to consider a change in hairstyle. Consult your hairstylist for advice.

Postpartum Blues and Depression

The postpartum period is filled with many adjustments and this can lead to the "baby blues" and, if it progresses, even to depression. There is intervention available and we will discuss this topic more in the chapter 20.

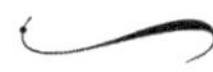

POSTPARTUM HAEMORRHAGE

Postpartum haemorrhage (PPH) is excessive blood lost that occurs after delivery. Most women can lose up to 500 ml of blood (about two cups) without any problems. This blood loss occurs as the placenta is separating from the uterine wall and from the site where the placenta was attached (the *placental bed*). As discussed earlier, the uterus contracts in order to seal off blood vessels and decrease bleeding; however, in some women this does not happen effectively, resulting in excessive blood loss.

Most cases of PPH occur in the first twenty-four hours after birth. If you have lost excessive blood, you may feel dizzy, short of breath, that your heart is racing, or even like you might collapse. Soaking more than one sanitary pad in two hours or less is also a concern. It is important to report any of these symptoms to your healthcare provider. You will likely still be in hospital if postpartum haemorrhage occurs early after delivery. The large amount of blood that flows to the baby during pregnancy still flows immediately after birth, which is why the sealing of the vessels is important. If your uterus does not contract well, it does not get firm and the vessels continue to bleed; this is called *uterine atony*. Other reasons include left-behind pieces of the placenta or an adherent placenta, an episiotomy or tears in the genital tract (vagina, cervix, or even uterus), and bleeding disorders.

Bleeding is an emergency situation, and your healthcare provider may place one hand in your vagina and one on your abdomen to massage your uterus to encourage it to contract, which may be uncomfortable. You will also be given medications called *uterotonics* to help your uterus contract. These medications can be given by injection or placed into the back passage (the anus).

Fluids will also be given through your veins to keep your blood pressure from falling too low (as a result of the blood loss), and a blood transfusion may be necessary to replace the blood that has been lost. The amount of blood you need will depend on your haemoglobin level. A catheter is placed in your bladder to ensure that you are excreting a sufficient amount of urine.

If the excessive bleeding is happening because of pieces of placenta left behind or the entire placenta is unable to be removed, you will have to go to the operating theatre to have it removed in a short procedure.

In some rare instances, the bleeding cannot be controlled by any of the ways described above, and you may need to be taken to the operating theatre wherein a stitch is placed around the uterus to encourage it to contract, or stiches are placed in some of the vessels that supply blood to the uterus in aims to decrease the bleeding. If all of this fails or your placenta is unable to be removed from its attachment site, the uterus may have to be removed in order to prevent death from uncontrollable bleeding.

Some hospitals and centres have a method called *uterine artery embolisation* where a special material (in the form of little pellets) is placed into some of the vessels supplying blood to the uterus with the guidance of an image displayed on the screen to ensure it is placed in the correct place. These pellets decrease the amount of blood flowing to the uterus.

Postpartum haemorrhage can also occur more than twenty-four hours after delivery to up to weeks after. This can be due to any of the reason mentioned earlier or due to infection. If infection of the uterus (*endometritis*) is diagnosed, you will be prescribed antibiotics for several days and medications to control the bleeding.

BREASTFEEDING AND BOTTLE-FEEDING

BREASTFEEDING

Breast milk is made of elements such as protein, vitamins, and carbohydrates that are essential for an infant's development. Breastfeeding may be exclusive or partial.

Breastfeeding should be commenced within one hour of delivery to maximize success. Although breastfeeding may be a challenge and getting the baby to latch on may feel unnatural at first, and this can frustrate a new mother, don't feel bad if you feel this way. Remember both you and the baby are learning. If you are breastfeeding, you need two hundred more calories per day and at least 1000 mg of calcium a day (this can be obtained from eating dairy products daily or calcium supplements).

Colostrum is the "first" milk. It is the clear or yellow substance that is produced in small quantities initially when you breastfeed. It is rich in substances that help to prevent infection. Breastfeeding should be "on demand," meaning whenever your baby is hungry (we will talk more about these hunger cues below). With time, you and your baby will develop a feeding schedule that fits his or her needs.

Benefits to the infant:

- Increased bonding with mother
- Improved development of the jaw muscles
- Protection against diseases such as diabetes and celiac disease (a disease of the gut in which there is an inability to digest gluten)
- Decreased risk of developing allergies, asthma, and eczema
- Decreased risk of diarrhea, lung infection, and ear infections
- Lowered risk of *necrotizing enterocolitis* (a disease in which part of the gut can die and stop functioning)

- Help in prevention of childhood obesity and childhood cancers, such as leukemia and lymphoma
- Decreased risk of sudden infant death
- Lowered risk of cardiovascular disease as an adult

Benefits to you:

- Helps prevent bleeding postpartum
- Helps womb return to normal state
- Facilitates weight loss postpartum
- Keeps period away, allowing you to increase your red blood count postdelivery
- Acts as a form of contraception
- Reduces risk of osteoporosis in future
- Decreases risk of cancer of the uterus, ovaries, and breast
- Saves money and makes travelling easier
- Reduces risk of type II diabetes

Preparing to breastfeed, what do I need?

- Two to three sleeping bras and a few nursing camisoles
- Nipple cream (apply before and after feeding to reduce the chance of sore nipples)
- Nursing pads (disposable or reusable)
- Nursing bras
- Possibly a breast pump (electrical or manual)
- Cold compress (to relieve sore nipples and pain)
- Hot compress (to relieve breast engorgement)

Can I take medications while breastfeeding?
Some medications are excreted in small amounts into your breast milk while others may become present in larger quantities. Contact your healthcare provider before taking any medications while breastfeeding.

Tips on improving latch

- Consider taking a class and watching videos. Some hospitals offer breastfeeding sessions before they discharge you and your baby.
- Get comfortable; consider using a recliner position and nursing pillows.
- Prepare and position your infant to latch on well, which allows baby's mouth to cover the areola (coloured area underneath the nipple) bottom and top.
- When your baby has a good latch, you will feel a tugging sensation on the breast and the baby's bottom lip should be curled out and his nose pointed upward. Sucking motions will usually become slow and rhythmic once a proper latch is established and flow is good.

When your milk comes in (called *let-down*), you may become engorged. This usually happens the first two to four days after delivery. The breasts become very firm and swollen, and you may experience pain, sometimes with a mild fever.

Breastfeeding multiples

You can breastfeed each infant one at a time or two at one time. There is no wrong way. The important thing is to make sure that you are comfortable and ensure that each infant gets sufficient time to nurse. We will talk more about this in the section on multiple gestation.

Breastfeeding while pregnant and tandem nursing

You may breastfeed during a subsequent pregnancy, but you should check with your healthcare provider first. You must make sure that you are eating a balanced diet. Be prepared that your nipples may be sore, that your milk supply may decrease, and that your morning sickness may be worsened by the breastfeeding.

As your tummy expands, you may have to find other positions to breastfeed. You may consider having the toddler kneel, stand, or lay on the side.

In the early days postdelivery, you may consider reserving the colostrum for the newborn, so nurse the newborn first. Consider getting to know other moms who are tandem nursing so that they can share some tips and advice on breastfeeding.

Lactation and fertility
Most mothers who are exclusively breastfeeding will remain infertile for six months. This is maintained by breastfeeding every three hours in the day and every six hours at night.

Engorgement
An engorged breast feels swollen and may be a bit firm. You may also have a fever until it is relieved. Some babies find it difficult to latch onto an engorged breast; expression of the milk ducts near the alveolar region makes it easier. The time while breasts are engorged can be a frustrating time for you and your baby; just be patient and continue breastfeeding. Engorgement usually does not last more than one to two days and can be prevented or relieved in the following ways:

- Nurse for at least fifteen to twenty minutes on each breast before switching breasts.
- Alternate the breast that you offer the baby first.
- Change the infant's position to allow complete emptying of the ducts of each breast.
- Use a breast pump or older toddler (if tandem nursing) to help relieve a plugged duct.
- Massage breasts manually with your hands to encourage expression.
- Use a heating pad to encourage flow or a cooling pad to decrease pain.
- Take a hot shower with the water directed towards the engorged breast.
- Make sure your nursing bra fits well.
- Protect your breasts.

Mastitis

This is inflammation and infection of the breast usually due to a blocked milk duct. The breast will be red, swollen, and painful, and you may also have a fever and not feel well. This condition is treated with antibiotics and expressing the breast milk. Standing under a hot shower can help with milk release. Your baby can also continue to breastfeed to aid in release of the blocked milk duct. Don't worry, your baby will not get the infection.

How do I know that my infant is eating enough?

- Soiling two to four diapers a day (breastfed babies can soil up to ten diapers a day)
- Wetting eight to twelve diapers a day
- Gaining 0.5 ounces a day in weight
- Acting satisfied after a meal (your baby will usually let go of the breast and be calm and relaxed)

As babies may pass urine and faeces together before a new diaper change, it may be difficult to count diapers based on one or the other separately. But generally, you should at least see four diapers soiled with feces in the diaper changes. Cues that your baby is still hungry include:

- Smacking and opening his mouth
- Turning the mouth towards the chest of whomever is holding her
- Sucking his fists and fingers (or anything that may get too near the mouth, such as clothing)
- Attempting to position herself for nursing
- Making little fussy noises while squirming about
- Crying and moving the head quickly from side to side (this is a late sign, so when possible feed at earlier cues).

Once your baby starts crying, you may need to calm him or her down in order for latching to be successful. Swaddling, rocking, or skin-to-skin contact are some techniques for calming, and you will learn what works best for your baby.

Storing Breast milk

Wash your hands before expressing breast milk. Your breast milk can be at room temperature (up to 80 degrees Fahrenheit) in a cool, dry area for up to eight hours, but it should not be left out for longer than this. Ideally it should be stored in clean, preferably sterilized, glass bottles, hard plastic bottles, or special breast milk storage bags that you can find at a baby store. The container should have a tight seal and the date when milk was expressed should be placed on them. Storage times for breast milk are outlined in table 2. Breast milk stored in the refrigerator should be placed in the back.

Table 2

BREAST MILK STORAGE TIME	
ROOM TEMPERATURE	
• **Up to 80°F**	4–8 hours
• **≥ 80°F**	3–4 hours
FRIDGE (≤ 40°F)	
• **Fresh Milk**	2 days
• **Thawed Milk**	24 hours
FRIDGE FREEZER	2 weeks
SEPARATE FREEZER	3 months
UPRIGHT DEEP FREEZER	6 months

Store in small "single-feed" quantities of about two to four ounces. This prevents wastage of your precious milk (as milk left over from a feed should be discarded after about an hour). When it is time to use the milk, thaw slowly in the fridge, in a container with cool water or under cool running water. Once thawed, you can use it. You should never refreeze thawed milk and never heat breast milk in the microwave or on the stove as this destroys the protective enzymes and antibodies. If you need to warm the milk, place the bottle or storage bag in a bowl of very warm water. You should not add freshly pumped milk to frozen milk.

Increasing your breast milk

Galactagogues are substances claimed to increase breast milk supply. *Prolactin* is a woman's main breast milk–producing hormone. Most medications that act as galactagogues work by increasing prolactin levels. Galactagogues are foods such as oatmeal, vitamins such as B-complex, herbs, or medications that can help to increase breast-milk supply. Different cultures have special foods that are thought to enhance milk production.

With proper support and information, most mothers are able to produce more than enough milk for their baby (or babies). However, if you think you have a low milk supply problem, it would be wise to talk to your healthcare provider and a lactation expert, to evaluate the issue, to decide if a galactagogue would be helpful in your case. Types of galactagogues include the following:

- *Domperidone* (Motilium®): a prescription drug used for gastrointestinal disorders; however, there is evidence that shows that domperidone is an effective galactagogue also with few side effects. But, it should be avoided if you have a history of heart problems.
- *Metoclopramide* (Maxolon®): another prescription drug used to treat gastrointestinal disorders. Metoclopramide can also be used to increase milk supply, but it has more side effects, especially on the nervous system, such as restlessness, drowsiness, fatigue, and depression.
- *Fenugreek*: enjoyed in many parts of the world as a culinary herb/ spice. Fenugreek has historically been used as a galactagogue for both human mothers and dairy animals around the world.

A galactagogue works best when a mother has low prolactin levels (i.e., when there is a truly low milk supply issue) and after a mother has received assessment, support, and education to improve her breastfeeding or expressing technique.

BOTTLE-FEEDING

Bottle-feeding is the alternative if you are unable to breastfeed. If this is your option, do not feel upset that you are depriving your baby of breast milk. Formulas created for babies supply all the necessary nutrients for your baby to thrive and be healthy. However, if you have no reason not to breastfeed, then you should, as breast milk provides more protective benefits than man-made formulas and is therefore preferred. With so many formulas available today, it can be confusing walking into the store. But below is some information to give you more clarity.

Types of Infant Formulas

- *Cow's milk–based:* these are made from cow's milk and contain lactose (a milk protein).
- *Soy-based:* these are made from soy protein. They can be used for infants who cannot tolerate lactose (lactose intolerant) or are allergic.
- *Special formulas:* reserved for babies that require a low-salt diet or who cannot digest whey and casein proteins found in other formulas.

Formulas can be powdered (which require mixing with sterilized water), liquid premixed (ready to eat), or liquid-concentrated (which must also be mixed with sterilized water). Sterilize water by bringing it to a boil in a clean container. Powdered formula is the least expensive.

Always follow the instructions on the container when using formula. Never add more or less water to formulas than suggested on the container as this can make your baby very sick, not grow well, have seizures, develop diarrhea, become dehydrated, and even die. There are many different brand names of formulas and any can be used, just always check the expiration date on the formula. Formula does not need to be heated before feeding, but if your baby prefers warm milk, you may do so, but never heat in a microwave.

You can also alternate breastfeeding with bottle-feeding. Some mothers who have to return to work or may have very demanding daily schedules can choose this option. Infants under six months do not need additional water as mixed formula and breast milk contains enough water for them.

CONTRACEPTION POSTPARTUM

You have just had a baby; the last thing you want to think about is getting pregnant again immediately. For this reason, most women want some method of contraception. There are two main methods: *reversible* and *permanent* contraception. Reversible contraception may be long-term or short-term.

If you have decided that your family number is complete or there is a medical reason why you should not have another baby then permanent contraception is the best choice. Two methods are *bilateral tubal ligation* (BTL) and Essure®.

BILATERAL TUBAL LIGATION AND ESSURE®

Bilateral tubal ligation (BTL) interrupts the fallopian tube, preventing an egg from reaching sperm. It can be done by an open procedure in which a small incision is made on the abdomen and the tubes are accessed through it. BTL may also be done laparoscopically, which uses a surgical instrument through a small, 1.5 cm to 2 cm, incision on the abdomen to reach the tubes guided by an image of the tubes projected on a display monitor. A band or clip can be placed on the tubes or a suture can be used to tie and cut the tubes, removing a portion.

Essure® is done with another surgical instrument called a *hysteroscope* (which is a little narrower than a sipping straw). It is inserted into the vagina,

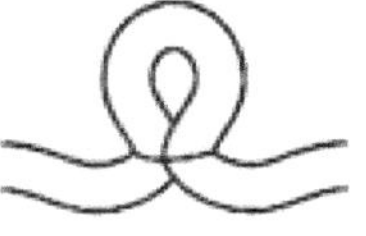

Figure 13. An example of tubal ligation

then cervix up to the opening of the tube inside the uterine cavity. The image is projected on a display monitor. A flexible coil is inserted to block the opening of the tubes, which prevents sperm from reaching the egg to fertilize it. This procedure can be done in an office in about five minutes and is usually not painful, but some women experience mild cramping after the procedure. The coil device does not become fully effective until three months after placement, so if you have gotten this form of contraception you must use backup protection for three months until it is confirmed the coil is effective. This confirmation can be done by a simple X-ray.

Vasectomy

Men can also play a part in contraception by having a procedure called a *vasectomy*. During this procedure the tube (called the *vas deferens*) running from the testes (located in the scrotal sac) that transport sperm to the penis is cut and tied, preventing sperm from being a part of the fluid that is ejaculated from the penis during sex. A man can still have an erection and orgasm after this procedure.

Long-Term Reversible Contraception

Most long-term reversible contraceptive methods are over 99 percent effective (when used correctly), and they include the following methods in table 3 below.

Table 3

Contraceptive Method	Type	How often Given	Effectiveness
IUD:	Copper T®	10 years	99%
	Mirena®	5 years	99%
	Skyla®	3 years	99%
Injectable Hormone:	Progestin Only	Monthly or every 3 months	97%
	Combination Progestin and Estrogen	Monthly	97%
Hormonal Implants:	Implanon®	3 years	99%
	Jadelle®	5 years	99%

If an intrauterine device (IUD) is left in place past the time it is to be used for, there is a risk of infection with a bacterium called *Actinomyces*. This can cause vaginal bleeding, discomfort in the pelvic region, and a vaginal discharge.

The injectable hormones are given into the muscle tissue of the upper arm or buttocks. Implants are placed just under the skin on the inside aspect of the upper arm and are small rods the size of a matchstick.

Hormonal contraception can cause breast tenderness, nausea, and vomiting in some women; however, this usually resolves in three to six months. Irregular or absent menses can also occur. Methods containing an estrogen can lead to *venous thromboembolism* and should be avoided if you have a blood-clotting disorder, smoke, or have had a blood clot in the past.

Estrogens can also decrease breast-milk supply so it is important that breastfeeding is well established if you are considering its use. It should be avoided within the first six weeks postpartum and, if possible, the first six months while breastfeeding.

SHORT-TERM REVERSIBLE CONTRACEPTION

- <u>Pill</u>: 92 percent effective
- <u>Patch</u>: 92 percent effective
- <u>Vaginal ring</u>: 92 percent effective
- <u>Vaginal sponge</u>: 85 percent effective in women who have never given birth, but 75 percent effective in women who have.
- <u>Cervical cap</u>: 85 percent effective
- <u>Diaphragm</u>: 85 percent effective.
- <u>Female condom</u>: 80 percent effective
- <u>Male condom</u>: 85 percent effective
- <u>Lactation Amenorrhoea Method (LAM)</u>: 98 percent effective
- <u>Natural Family Planning</u>: 96 percent effective
- <u>Coitus Interruptus:</u> 75 to 80 percent effective

These methods can be used if you only want to prevent pregnancy for a short time or only during fertile days during the cycle. However, these methods can be used for as long as contraception is required.

Birth Control Pill

The birth control pill can be a combination of progestin or estrogen or progestin only (known as the *minipill*). The pill (as with other estrogen-containing methods) should not be taken sooner than six weeks after delivery because it can lead to a greater chance of a blood clot. Also because it has estrogen, it should be avoided in breastfeeding moms. The minipill is perfectly suited for breastfeeding moms; in fact, it may even increase your breast milk production. It contains twenty-eight hormone pills and must be taken every day at the same time. Failure to do this can cause you to become pregnant. Overall, six women out of one hundred women can get pregnant each year even when the pill is taken correctly.

The combined pill pack has twenty-one pills, one per day, followed by seven *dummy pills*. You will have a period during those last seven days. Some packs use iron pills as the dummy pills. This can be very useful in helping you to build up your iron levels after having a baby or just replacing the iron that is lost in the blood during your period.

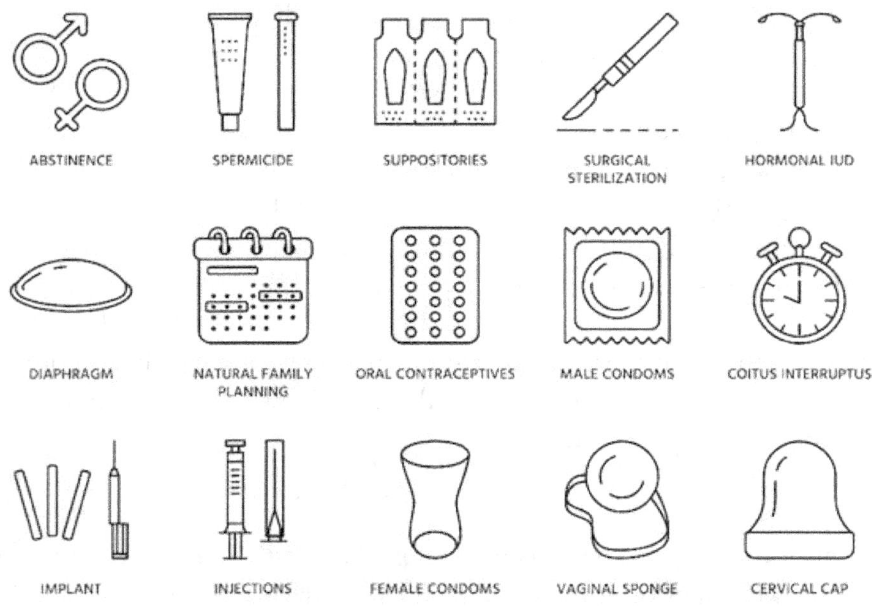

Figure 14. Contraceptive methods

Patch and Vaginal Ring
Both of these devices release progestin and an estrogen. The patch is a small sticky bandage placed on the arm, abdomen, back, or hips. It is placed on the skin for three weeks out of every month and then removed for one week; a new one is placed again the following month. The vaginal ring is placed in the vagina with the same timing as the patch. The week that both devices are not in place, you will have your period.

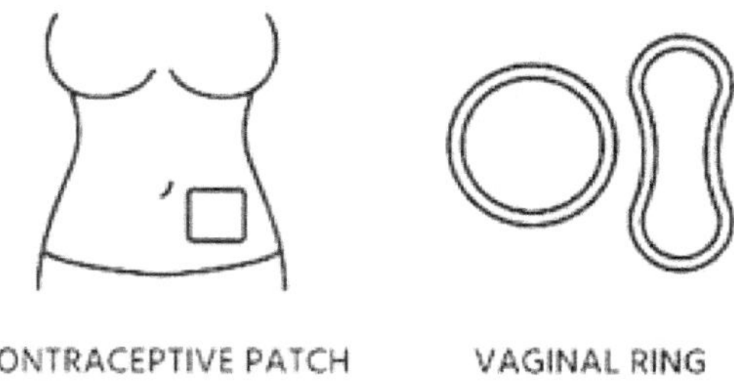

Figure 15. The patch and ring

Cap, Diaphragm, and Sponge

These devices are not used as much as other types of contraception. Some women find them more tedious to use and would rather a method that does not need frequent removing and replacing. All of these methods are placed in the vagina and cover the cervix and are used before having sex. The cap must be fitted by your healthcare provider. The cap and diaphragm may not fit as snugly over the cervix as they do when not pregnant and therefore can be less effective just after delivery. These methods should be used with a *spermicide*, which is a chemical placed in the vagina that destroys sperm. Spermicide is hardly ever used alone because it may not destroy all the sperm. They come in several forms: cream, foam, jelly or suppositories.

Female Condom

This is another method that is not used a lot. A female condom is a plastic tube-like structure that on one end has a cap that covers the cervix and the tubing lines the vagina up to the opening of the vagina.

Male Condom

The male condom is made of a rubber-like material that is placed over the erected male penis just prior to sex. Condoms have an added benefit in protecting against sexually transmitted infections, such as HIV, chlamydia, gonorrhoea, and other STIs. The condom catches the sperm at the tip of the condom, preventing it from entering the vagina.

Lactation Amenorrhoea Method (LAM)
This method occurs naturally with frequent breastfeeding. Breastfeeding causes release of the hormone *prolactin* that prevents release of hormones that would allow production of eggs in your ovaries. This method is only effective if:

1. Your period has not returned.
2. You are breastfeeding on demand:
   a. at least every three hours.
   b. with no supplemental infant feeding (as this decreases the frequency of breastfeeding).
3. Six months has not passed since the birth of your baby.

Once none of the above has occurred, this method is more than 98 percent effective in preventing pregnancy.

Natural Family Planning, Absitnence and Coitus Interruptus
These methods are associated with higher failure rates when compared to other methods (due to conscious "breaking of the rules"). Complete absitnence is not a feasible option for most couples, however, periodic abstinence may be agreed upon. In natural family planning the female must have regular menstrual cycles and refrain from sexual intercourse during the fertile period. She may also observe changes in the cervical mucous (mucous becomes clear and stretchy during the fertile period and is thick, opaque or absent otherwise). When this method is used perfectly every time, it has an effectiveness as high as 96%. Coitus interruptus requires removal of the penis from the vagina prior to ejaculation of semen. It is important to note that sperm can be released in the vagina even prior to removal of the penis, therefore failure of this method is high, with an efficacy of 75-80%. This method requires good self-control in the male and can reduce the pleasure of intercourse. This method was used for centuries before other methods became available. A man concerned about "discarding" his precious seed may be reminded about the

Bible story of Onan in Genesis 38:8–10. The family dynamics of that story, however, is quite different from Christian families today. All three of these methods decribed may prove difficult to use in the postpartum period given the normal physical changes that take place in the body during this time.

SECTION 3
HIGH-RISK PREGNANCIES, DISEASES, AND OTHER COMPLICATIONS

The LORD will give you prosperity in the land he swore to your ancestors to give you, blessing you with many children.

—Deuteronomy 28:11 (NLT)

C H A P T E R   6

MONITORING FETAL HEALTH DURING PREGNANCY

THERE ARE VARIOUS modalities used throughout pregnancy and in the intrapartum period to monitor the well-being of your baby. These tests help your healthcare provider to make the best decisions to ensure the best outcome possible for your baby. They may indicate when something is not going well with your baby, allowing for intervention, or they may indicate that everything is going well. These tests can easily be done and do not harm you or your baby. They are done at or after 28 weeks (except Doppler velocimetry, which can be done earlier).

NONSTRESS TEST

This test is noninvasive and monitors your baby's heartbeat (in association with its movement) over twenty to forty minutes and traces it out on a special paper. Your baby should have an increase in its heart rate every time he or she moves, and this is outlined on the paper. If the baby does not move, it may mean that the baby is sleeping, so the test may be repeated later or done for longer than twenty minutes. It is called nonstress because your baby is not under any stress when the test is done. Contractions would be considered a stress.

WHY WOULD THIS TEST BE PERFORMED?

- You are past your due date.
- Your pregnancy is considered "high risk."
- Your baby is not moving as often as before.

This test can tell if there is insufficient oxygen getting to your baby from your blood supply. Certain conditions can cause this to happen. Also the test can be abnormal if the umbilical cord is being compressed or if the baby is in any other type of distress.

ULTRASOUND

Doppler Velocimetry

We spoke about ultrasound earlier; however, that time the reason for performing an ultrasound was a little different. Ultrasound in this instance measures the speed and direction of the blood flow in the vessels in the placenta, particularly from baby to mother through the two umbilical arteries. The flow depends on how well your baby's heart is pumping blood and how healthy the placenta is. This ultrasound machine technology calculates this flow and gives it a number called the *resistance index* that can be interpreted by your doctor. Blood flow from the baby to the placenta removes waste gases out of the fetus (e.g., carbon dioxide). If flow in the umbilical artery is impeded in any way, your baby can become hypoxic (meaning deprived of adequate oxygen supply) and not receive enough nutrients. This can lead to poor growth and even death if it occurs for over a long period of time or is severe.

There are certain conditions that you may have or the baby may have in which this test is performed, including:

- Intrauterine growth restriction
- Rhesus isoimmunisation
- High blood pressure and diabetes
- Low amniotic fluid

Biophysical Profile

This test includes:

- Measuring the amount of amniotic fluid around your baby
- Counting how frequently your baby breathes
- Observing the way your baby moves

A nonstress test may also be included.

Now, before we go on, I know you are wondering how your baby can breathe in amniotic fluid! Well, the baby moves its breathing (respiratory) muscles and inhales and exhales, but no oxygen is going into the lungs; your baby is just going through the motions. This tells us that the nervous system of the baby it working well enough to tell the respiratory muscles to move every so often.

The biophysical profile is given a score, which your healthcare provider uses to determine if your baby is well or not. This test is done after 28 weeks and takes about thirty minutes to perform. A score of eight to ten means your baby is healthy, six means the test needs to be repeated in several hours, and a score of four or less means your baby is not well and needs to be delivered. Other tests may be done along with the biophysical profile in order for your provider to make a well-informed decision regarding when and how you should be delivered.

FETAL KICK COUNTS

In some high-risk pregnancies or when you are not feeling your baby move as often, you may be asked to do a fetal kick count. This test is dependent on your consistency. You will be asked to take a moment during the day when your baby is most active and when you are not distracted to count the amount of times your baby moves. Get in a comfortable spot, as you are going to be there for two hours. Your baby should move at least ten times within two hours. If you notice it is less, contact your healthcare provider immediately.

CONTRACTION STRESS TEST

This test is similar to the nonstress test, but it is done under "stress." Remember we said that contractions are considered a stress. Two probes are attached to your abdomen to record the fetal heart rate and contractions. Contractions are stimulated using a dilute amount of synthetic oxytocin, or you may be asked to massage your nipples. The test helps to determine if your baby can tolerate the repeated contractions that occur during labour without experiencing decreased oxygen supply. Normally during a contraction, your baby's oxygen levels drop for a short period of time. A healthy fetus can deal with this very well; however, some babies have a slowing of their heart rate, which results in poor blood flow.

CHAPTER 7

PRETERM PRELABOUR RUPTURE OF THE MEMBRANES AND PRETERM LABOUR AND DELIVERY

PRETERM PRELABOUR RUPTURE of the membranes (also called preterm *premature* rupture of the membranes) is a condition in which the amniotic sac breaks before 37 weeks but at or after 24 weeks. As discussed earlier, the amniotic sac helps to form a protective barrier for the fetus within the uterus. When it is lost this increases the risk of infection to the fetus if bacteria, which may be normal in the vagina, gets into the uterus by moving upward. This is called *chorioamnionitis*. If this occurs your baby will have to be delivered, because infection within the womb is not tolerated well by the fetus and may lead to death of the baby and infection in the blood of the mother (which if severe enough can lead to death in the mother or possible admission to the intensive care unit).

More than 50 percent of women will spontaneously go into labour when their water breaks. If this does not occur within the first twenty-four hours to one week, the pregnancy may be prolonged to allow your baby's lungs to mature. Labour that occurs before 37 weeks is called *preterm labour*.

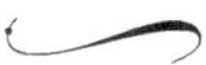

FREQUENTLY ASKED QUESTIONS
What Causes Preterm Prelabour Rupture of Membranes?
Several factors can contribute to this early breaking of the waters:

- Infection with chlamydia, gonorrhoea, or trichomonas
- The presence of a bacteria in the vagina such as group B streptococcus or bacterial vaginosis, and in the urine (i.e., urinary tract infection)
- Kidney infections
- Dental infections
- Infection in the uterus
- If it occurred in a previous pregnancy
- Twin pregnancy (or more)
- Excessive amniotic fluid (*polyhydramnios*)
- Trauma to the abdomen (being hit in the abdomen)

When the water breaks, it may be complicated by the cord dropping out or into the vagina (which is an emergency requiring delivery right away). Also placental abruption can occur leading to the need for urgent delivery (we will talk about this condition in chapter 14).

What If My Amniotic Sac Breaks and I Do Not Go into Labour?

You and the baby will be monitored using ultrasound, some tests of fetal well-being, checking pulse and temperature, and a blood test. If any of these tests suggest there is an infection or the baby is in trouble, you will have to be delivered. Otherwise you will also be given an injection of a medication called *dexamethasone* or *betamethasone* to help stimulate the baby's lungs to mature. Also, a medication called *magnesium sulphate* may be given if you are less than 32 weeks to help protect the baby's brain from damage. Antibiotics will be used for about seven days to help prevent infection from occurring (although it can still occur even with them). You will most likely be admitted to hospital until the baby is delivered; however, depending on the situation, some women may be allowed home with very close monitoring. You and your healthcare provider must decide if you are able to have this form of treatment outside of hospital.

The aim is to prolong the pregnancy until the lungs are mature, this is around 34 weeks for most pregnancies. If you are a diabetic, your baby's lungs may take a bit longer to mature. A special test can be done on the amniotic fluid to determine this, as lung maturity can occur as early as 32 weeks. If this test is not available in your area, you will usually be delivered at 34 to 36 weeks as the lungs are mature by then, so there is no need to keep the baby in the uterus any longer as the risk of infection goes up the longer you are pregnant after this time. Your baby will most likely have to be admitted to the neonatal intensive care unit for some time, but once the baby is born the paediatrician can fully assess the baby and keep you up to date on his or her progress.

WILL MY BABY SURVIVE IF IT IS DELIVERED EARLY?

This all depends on how early you deliver and where you deliver. Some countries have medical equipment in place that can support the baby outside the womb as young as 23 weeks gestation. Other areas, however, may not be able to that early and the chance of survival is less, and even at later gestational ages survival can vary from place to place. Generally speaking, however, there is a 90 to 100 percent chance of survival of your baby after 34 weeks (this may be less if other complications are present). The neonatologist at the hospital where you are admitted can give you information on the rates of survival that is expected for your baby.

WHAT IF MY WATER BREAKS AT 23 WEEK OR EVEN 22 WEEKS?

When it happens at this gestational age, a discussion needs to be made with your healthcare provider concerning the likelihood of the great risk of infection over the benefit of trying to prolong the pregnancy. The fetus needs amniotic fluid for the lungs to mature and for the limbs to keep moving around in the uterus. The lungs are very far from fully mature at this time, and the loss of fluid can cause underdeveloped lungs (*lung hypoplasia*), which can cause problems that include lifelong lung disease in your child or even death before delivery. The lack of fluid can also cause the baby's limbs to become stiff, and when the baby is born they are unable to move the limbs well; they stay in the position they were in while in the womb, this is called *limb contractures*. At less than 22 weeks the baby's eyes are usually still fused shut and are unable to open if delivered at this stage.

What About Preterm Labour?

The cause of preterm labour is similar to that for prelabour rupture of the membranes. However, because the amniotic sac is still intact, it is treated differently. Labour can be stopped with certain medications to allow prolongation of the pregnancy and allow full maturity of your baby. Sometimes these medications do not help, and you deliver a preterm baby. Preterm babies often have to be admitted to the neonatal intensive care unit. Other babies may do very well after birth, and if they have attained a particular weight may be allowed home with you on discharge from the hospital.

If you start feeling contractions early in your pregnancy or your water breaks, contact your healthcare provider immediately.

COPING WITH AN INFANT IN THE NEONATAL INTENSIVE CARE UNIT (NICU) OR SPECIAL CARE BABY UNIT (SCBU)

Having your baby go to NICU or special care can be jarring. Especially when you had anticipated taking your infant home with you. An infant that is born early or has complications at the time of delivery may warrant the additional care or interventions provided in these special settings, however.

This time may be an emotional rollercoaster as you experience different emotions throughout the process. Focus on the positive and continue to speak life over your infant.

Remember not to neglect yourself or your partner. Events such as sleeping and keeping yourself groomed will enable you to have the energy to make it through. Encourage the father as well, because even though he may not show it, he could be experiencing the same emotions as you are regarding the baby. Also know that you may feel differently at different times.

Spend time with your infant and remember he or she belongs to you. Take time to learn your infant's habits, touch your infant, and dress your infant if possible. Remember that your baby is aware and is developing. Consider posting a picture of you and the father, if allowed, in your baby's space.

Keep track of your baby's progress. Document his or her milestones and weights.

Pump, pump, and pump some more. Whether you had planned to breast-feed or not, breast milk will do wonders for your infant while he or she is thriving in the NICU or SCBU. It will contain many nutrients that may be lifesaving. Be patient and stay hydrated. When you pump, it may not seem like much may come at first, but remember that every drop counts.

Do not neglect the power of prayer. More than ever this is a time to communicate with God and give Him thanks and praise.

C H A P T E R   8

MULTIPLE GESTATION

MULTIPLE GESTATION REFERS to any pregnancy in which there is more than one fetus present. The most common type of multiples is twins, but there are also triplets, quadruplets, quintuplets, sextuplets, septuplets, and octuplets. Greater than eight have been documented, but no live births have resulted from these pregnancies to date. Twins can be identical (*monozygotic*, 40 percent) or nonidentical (*dizygotic*, 60 percent). Rarely twins can be joined together at different locations on the body; this condition is called *conjoined twins* and occurs in less than 1 percent of twin pregnancies.

Nonidentical twins tend to run in families and are more common in older women, Afro-Caribbean lineage (and other groups with African ancestry), having twins in a prior pregnancy, and a woman with five or more children. Generally twins occur one in every eighty births; however, the incidence has increased in recent years due to the use of in vitro fertilisation and drugs that stimulate ovulation (*ovulation induction*).

Nonidentical twins have separate amniotic sacs and placentas, which is referred to as a *dichorionic diamniotic gestation*. Identical twins can have separate sacs and placentas also or share the same sac (*monoamniotic*) and placenta (*monochorionic*) (See figure 16). You may hear your doctor refer to the pregnancy using these terms. The number of sacs and placentas are determined using ultrasound. If an ultrasound is done very early in the pregnancy (e.g., at 4 or 5 weeks), multiples may be missed and not seen until a later ultrasound.

It is very exciting for most families to be expecting multiples. It must be noted, however, that multiples are considered a high-risk pregnancy that can be associated with complications (see table 4 below). Your physician may,

102

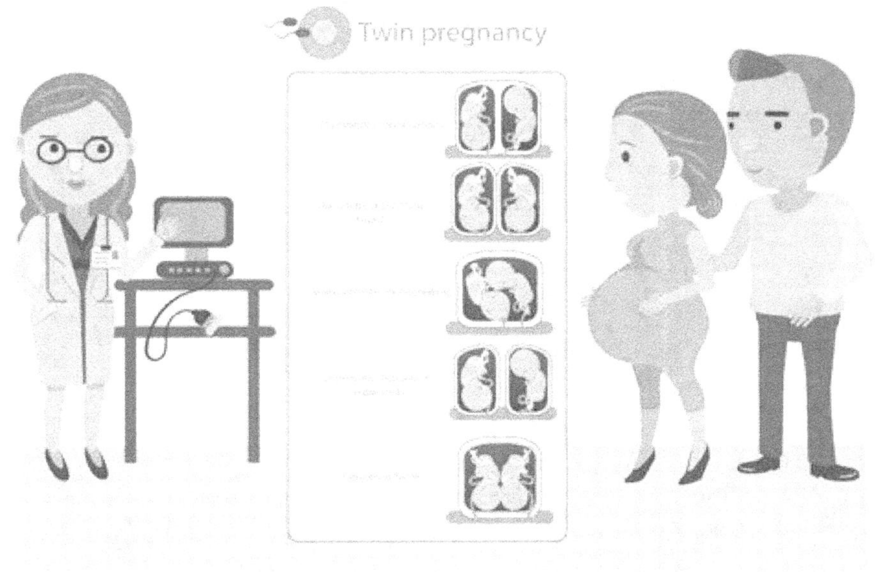

Figure 16. Twin Pregnancy

therefore, schedule more frequent visits, tests, and ultrasounds during your pregnancy. It is important that women receive iron supplementation of at least 30–60 mg a day and 5 mg folic acid.

Table 4: Potential Complications of Multiples

FOR THE FETUS	**FOR THE MOTHER**
Miscarriage	High blood pressure
Preterm labour and delivery	Diabetes in pregnancy (gestational diabetes)
Low birth weight	Need for caesarean section
Death of one or more of the babies	Nausea and vomiting
Abnormalities in development	Skin lesions/rash (especially on the abdomen and trunk.)

If other children are in the home, it is important to prepare them for the babies as it is not uncommon for there to be sibling rivalry or jealousy and even additional strain on a marriage. In all of this, it is good to recall two very relevant scriptures:

"Children are a gift from the LORD, they are a reward from him."

—PSALM 127:3 (NLT)

"For my strength is made perfect in weakness."

—2 CORINTHIANS 12:9C (KJV)

Most twins deliver spontaneously at around 35 weeks gestation. Triplets and quadruplets deliver at an average of 32 and 29 weeks respectively. At less than 34 weeks, most babies' lungs are not fully developed and require additional care in the NICU after birth. Preterm babies are also at risk for infections, feeding problems, vision problems, and bleeding within the brain that can lead to cerebral palsy or seizures.

The route of delivery of multiples will depend on how they are lying in the womb, any present complications, and how many weeks pregnant you are. The safest route will be chosen by your healthcare provider specific to your pregnancy; however, most pregnancies with triplets or greater will be delivered by caesarean section. Twins that are in the same sac (monoamniotic) should always be delivered by caesarean section at about 32 to 34 weeks to decrease the chances of the umbilical cords of the babies becoming entangled (which can lead to death within the uterus). If the first twin (that is, the twin closest to the cervix) is in the cephalic (head down) position, vaginal delivery is possible. If the first twin is breech (or not lying longitudinally) or the second twin is very small, caesarean section is usually the safest route. Otherwise the second twin can be delivered by breech extraction (where the physician will gently hold on to the baby's feet and pull them out to the vagina and allow the delivery to continue.

Having support after the delivery of twins is very beneficial to the mother to decrease stress and the risk of postpartum depression.

Breastfeeding is possible with twins but becomes technically difficult (and possibly tiresome) with more than three babies. It is a misconception that milk supply is not adequate for multiples; in fact, the more frequent the breast is emptied of milk the greater the supply. Pumping breast milk is always an alternative. It is a bit of a cliché, but still very true that "breast is best!" Suggested breastfeeding techniques for twins include the following types of holds:

- *Double football hold:* both babies are held under each arm (like one would a football) and the head is placed at the breast.
- *Double cradle hold:* both babies are held in a cradling position with one baby at each breast with their bodies stretched across each arm, parallel to each other.
- *Criss-cross cradle hold (Front-cross):* both babies are cradled, but stacked one on top of the other in an "x" position.
- *Football and cradle hold:* a combination of the football and cradle method, one for each baby.
- *Upright hold (Upright latch or Saddle hold):* both babies are held in an upright position at each breast. This works best with older babies that have good head control.

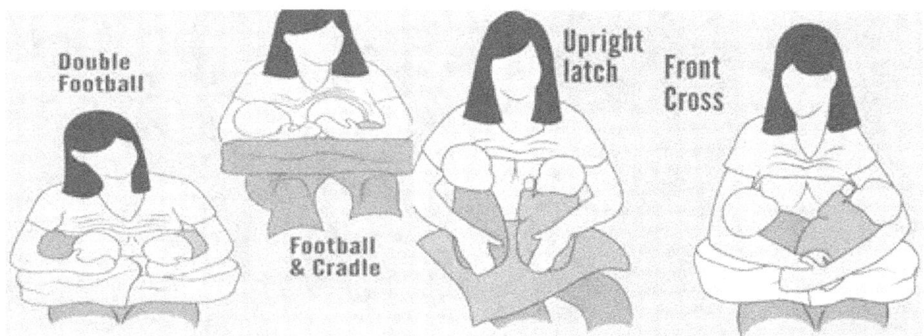

Figure 17. Examples of breastfeeding positions

Care for multiples should ideally occur in a tertiary-level institution where neonatal intensive care facilities are available.

Now, a little quiz for you!

Do you know the names of the first and second recorded twins in the Bible?

"When her days to give birth were completed, behold, there were twins in her womb."

—Genesis 25:24[2] (ESV)

"When the time of her labor came, there were twins in her womb. And when she was in labor, one put out a hand, and the midwife took and tied a scarlet thread on his hand, saying, 'This one came out first.' But as he drew back his hand, behold, his brother came out."

—Genesis 38:27–30[3] (ESV)

---

2 *Esau and Jacob*

3 *Perez and Zerah*

C H A P T E R   9

UTERINE FIBROIDS

FIBROIDS ARE NONCANCEROUS abnormal growths of muscular tissue that occur within the uterus. They are quite common among women, particularly women of black ethnicity. Up to 50 percent of women are without symptoms (*asymptomatic*), but at times troublesome symptoms occur resulting in frequent visits to the gynaecologist.

Fibroids occur most commonly in the reproductive age group (twenty to forty-nine years old) and they tend to decrease in size after menopause (around fifty-one years old). It has been observed that up to 80 percent of black women have fibroids, and they can be quite large, numerous, and diagnosed at an earlier age when compared to other ethnicities. In a percentage of women, it may have a genetic link, meaning it runs in families. Physicians are not fully clear on how fibroids start to grow, but we do know that their growth is accelerated by the female hormones estrogen and progesterone.

Symptoms of fibroids may be quite alarming to some women, as bleeding from the vagina is mostly frequently encountered. This bleeding can be a prolongation of a period, an extremely heavy period, or irregular heavy periods (and periods may also become painful). This pattern of bleeding can lead to dizziness, fatigue, heart palpitations, and a sudden loss of consciousness. One should seek immediate help at a physician's office or a hospital's emergency department should these symptoms occur. Acute pain from an inflammatory breaking down (degeneration) or the twisting of the fibroid can occur. If fibroids are very large, some women may notice an increase in the size of the abdomen, pelvic pressure, frequent urination, or an inability to pass stools. Fibroids can be deep within the muscle of the uterus (intramural), close to the inner lining of the uterus (submucosal), hanging from a stalk (pedunculated) or close to the outer surface (subserosal).

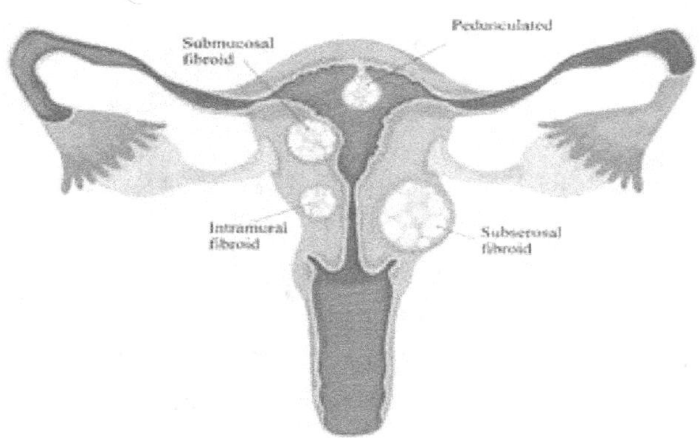

Figure 18: Uterine Fibroids

Only your physician can diagnose fibroids through asking you questions, a full physical examination (including a vaginal/pelvic exam), and an ultrasound of the reproductive organs (pelvic ultrasound). Blood tests are also done to assess for anemia (low haemoglobin levels).

There are several options for treating fibroids, and the method chosen will depend on your age, desire for children, and the availability of a particular treatment modality. A full discussion of the options should occur with your physician. Treatment is not the same for everyone, it must be individualized.

Treatment can be with the use of hormonal medications, in which the purpose is to reduce the abnormal pattern of vaginal bleeding and control pain. These medications include (most commonly) the combined oral contraceptive pill (the birth control pill), a levonorgestrel IUD, and the synthetic hormone *leuprolide*, among others.

Medications merely treat symptoms (i.e., they do not get rid of the fibroids), but it may be all that some women require. However, many women find that definitive treatment is needed in the form of surgery. The surgical options include removal of the fibroids (*myomectomy*), destruction of the fibroids using a specialized ultrasound beam, destruction of the fibroids using heat during laparoscopy (*radiofrequency thermal ablation*), occlusion of blood vessels connected to the fibroids feeding its growth (*uterine embolisation*), or removal of the womb (*hysterectomy*). These methods are available to alleviate symptoms and improve one's quality of life. There is no need for women to be ashamed or suffer.

I JUST FOUND OUT I HAVE FIBROIDS; HOW WILL THIS AFFECT MY PREGNANCY?

Before addressing this question, as noted prior, your chances of becoming pregnant may be decreased by the presence of fibroids. In some instances your physician may suggest removal of the fibroids if you have had difficulty conceiving, but that is dependent on the size and location of the fibroids. Other issues that may be affecting your fertility must also be addressed.

- Fibroids can lead to miscarriage in the first trimester and further on can lead to early (preterm) delivery.
- Episodes of pain from degenerating fibroids, requiring hospital treatment, may occur.
- Fibroids that are located in the lower part of the womb can result in a difficult labour. If they block the cervix, the baby is unable to makes its exit out of the womb at vaginal delivery. Fibroids may also cause the fetus to acquire an abnormal position within the womb (*malpresentation*), and in both the latter and former instances a caesarean section would be indicated.
- The muscles of the uterus contract after delivery of the placenta to decrease the amount of blood loss. When this normal muscle is replaced with fibroid tissue, it does not contract as well and may result in excessive blood loss after delivery (postpartum haemorrhage).
- Fibroids cannot be removed during pregnancy, as it would disrupt the pregnancy and result in loss of the baby. (Removal, if required, can be scheduled at a later time months after the pregnancy).

We know what you may be thinking, "Information overload; now I am even more nervous and fearful than before!" A full discussion can be made with your obstetrician. Seek medical care if you experience any of the symptoms above or just want further information on the topic. But we want to reassure you that fibroids are common in women, and many women have successful pregnancies even when they are present. The Word of God can provide reassurance also:

"So do not fear, for I am with you; do not be dismayed for I am your God. I will strengthen you and help you; I will uphold you with my righteous right hand."

—Isaiah 41:10 (NIV)

C H A P T E R   1 0

CARDIAC DISEASES

THE HEART IS the organ in the body that is responsible for carrying blood and oxygen around the mother's body as well as to and from the fetus. In pregnancy the amount of blood pumped by the heart increases by almost half, and therefore the heart (and its many different compartments, valves, and vessels) has to work a little harder.

Some maternal cardiac diseases carry a very low risk to the mother and the fetus. These include *mitral regurgitation, aortic regurgitation, hypertrophic cardiomyopathy, mitral valve prolapse,* and intracardiac shunts such as *atrial septal defects* and *ventricular septal defects.* If a mother (or father) was born with a heart disease (called *congenital heart disease*), the baby is at risk for having a congenital heart disease as well.

VALVE DEFECTS

Mitral valve prolapse is often well tolerated during pregnancy, and the prolapse may actually decrease because of the normal changes that the mother's heart goes through during pregnancy. Women with *pulmonic valve disease* and *tricuspid valve disease* may also have relatively uncomplicated pregnancies. But, some types of valve disorders may present problems with pregnancy.

Two such disorders are *mitral* or *aortic stenosis* (where the related valve is narrowed). Often these valve disorders are the result of rheumatic heart disease. If you have this, you may require additional visits to your doctor, medications, and specialized monitoring during labour and delivery. Your obstetric healthcare provider will liaison with a cardiologist and medical internist during your care and may even suggest that you have a valve replacement or have

111

the narrowed valve widened (*balloon valvotomy*) before conceiving. The reason for this is as pregnancy advances to the second and third trimesters, there is a high likelihood of heart failure and even death.

PULMONARY HYPERTENSION

Complications like pulmonary hypertension (elevated lung pressures), either due to congenital heart disease, lung disease, or connective tissue diseases (such as *systemic lupus erythematosus*), have a very high risk of death during pregnancy. Women who continue to have cyanosis (low blood oxygen) despite surgery are at high risk for maternal complications, premature delivery, small babies, blood clots in the vessels, and death during pregnancy. If you have poor cardiac function prior to the pregnancy, you may be unable to withstand the cardiac changes associated with pregnancy (e.g., increased blood volume) and therefore develop symptoms. If you have heart symptoms at rest, you are also among the highest at-risk populations for developing complications as pregnancy progresses.

ARRHYTHMIAS

Arrhythmias (irregular heart rhythms) may occur for the first time or occur with increased frequency during pregnancy. In women with structurally normal hearts, these arrhythmias usually do not pose a significant risk. However, the cause of the arrhythmia should be sought and treated appropriately. For women that develop atrial fibrillation, it is important to look for the underlying heart problem causing the atrial fibrillation. Atrial fibrillation is usually associated with valvular heart disease, hyperthyroidism, pulmonary embolism, or hypertension.

CARDIOMYOPATHY

Cardiac problems may arise during pregnancy in women who have had no history of cardiac problems. For example, heart failure (fluid overload) may occur because the increased volume of pregnancy is not tolerated. These women may have developed heart failure due to an underlying valvular disease, arrhythmia, and/or cardiomyopathy. A small number of women will develop a cardiomyopathy, a specific weakening of the heart muscle that appears to be caused by the pregnancy. This form of cardiomyopathy may occur at either the end of pregnancy or several months after delivery. It is not clear why this happens, and women may not have a complete recovery and/or the cardiomyopathy may reoccur with future pregnancies. Therefore, future childbearing would be contraindicated.

MYOCARDIAL INFARCTION

Although quite rare, women may present with a myocardial infarction (heart attack) during pregnancy. These women need to be assessed and treated as if they are not pregnant. Although certain drug choices can be made to decrease the risk to the fetus, management strategies are similar to the nonpregnant state, though certain precautions may be advised.

A successful pregnancy for women with heart disease requires specialized care, preconception evaluation, continuation of select medications, and close observation during the pregnancy.

> *"My flesh and my heart may fail, but God is the strength of my heart and my portion forever."*
>
> —PSALM 73:26 (NIV)

CHAPTER 11

HYPERTENSION

HYPERTENSION CAN BE present before pregnancy (although sometimes undiagnosed), or it can occur during pregnancy, which is known as *gestational hypertension* and *preeclampsia*. Preeclampsia being the most potentially life-threatening of them all.

Generally speaking, hypertension (also known as high blood pressure) is a condition in which the blood flowing through the arteries are under increased pressure, and this can result in damage to the lining of the vessels, particularly in sensitive organs such as the brain, heart, kidneys, eyes, and vessels in the legs. When it occurs in pregnancy, the mother is at risk for even further complications, and the fetus is also at risk.

PREECLAMPSIA

This condition includes high blood pressure, fluid retention, and spilling of proteins in the urine. It causes changes in your blood vessels that can affect multiple organs. Preeclampsia only occurs during pregnancy (after 20 weeks gestation) and can cause much harm to you or your baby. Most cases occur in the third trimester. Some pregnant women with this condition have no symptoms, or may only have symptoms when the condition has become suddenly severe, resulting in a poor outcome. During a routine antenatal visit, your healthcare provider may be able to detect the condition before symptoms occur. This is why it is important not to miss your appointments. In preeclampsia, your blood pressure is greater than or equal to a systolic (top number) of 140 or a diastolic (bottom number) of 90, which would be written as 140/90, and a urine sample reveals proteins in your urine. Many cases will present with symptoms that you may notice, which include:

- Nausea and vomiting
- Blurring of your vision, or seeing spots or flashing lights in your visual field
- Headaches around the front of the head
- Pain in the abdomen
- Swelling of your face or hands
- Rapid weight gain of more than four pounds a week

The ultimate cure for this condition is delivery. If preeclampsia occurs very early in your pregnancy, your doctor may be able to delay delivery for a while to allow the baby's lungs to mature in order to give the baby a better chance of survival. Delay of delivery usually is only necessary if you are less than 34 weeks. However, if complications of preeclampsia have already occurred in you or your fetus when you are diagnosed, delivery cannot be delayed. Severe cases of preeclampsia can cause your baby to not grow well, receive decreased amount of oxygen, and decrease the amount of amniotic fluid. It can lead to seizures (eclampsia), stroke, heart failure, fluid in the lungs, problems with the clotting of your blood, and (rarely) your liver tearing on the inside or changes in your vision. While awaiting the right time to deliver your baby, your healthcare provider will perform blood tests, start medications to help lower your blood pressure and prevent you from having a seizure, and give medications (*antenatal corticosteroids*) to help the lungs of your baby to mature if you are less than 34 weeks. A nonstress test and an ultrasound may also be done. Every pregnant mother is different, so you and your healthcare provider will work together to help attain the best outcome possible.

ECLAMPSIA

Eclampsia is seizures occurring in pregnancy. It does not include seizures that occur because of epilepsy. Preeclampsia can lead to eclampsia, or eclampsia can occur even before the symptoms of preeclampsia manifest. Unlike preeclampsia, eclampsia means delivery has to occur immediately (once the mother is stable), and for a patient that is not in active labour, the quickest route is via a caesarean section.

Patients do not know when they are having a seizure, nor do they remember the event. Immediately after a seizure the mother is drowsy and may sometimes be a bit aggressive; this will go away several minutes after. During a seizure the muscles of the body violently shake and become rigid, the eyes roll backward, and there may be tongue-biting and loss of control of bladder function. In hospital, magnesium sulphate is given to stop the seizure and prevent others. If a seizure happens at home, the person with you should turn you on your left side. Nothing should be placed in your mouth! This could lead to choking. The emergency medical service should be called immediately for transport to the hospital. Both preeclampsia and eclampsia are serious complications of pregnancy, and both can show up for the first time after delivery (usually within the first 48 hours).

WHO CAN GET PREECLAMPSIA AND ECLAMPSIA?

Any pregnant women can get this condition. However, your risk is higher if:

- it occurred in a previous pregnancy;
- siblings or your mother had it;
- you have diabetes, kidney disease, or lupus;
- you are obese;
- you are black (Afro-Caribbean or African American), Latino, Mediterranean, or a Pacific Islander;
- you are younger than twenty or older than thirty-five; or
- you have chronic hypertension or gestational hypertension.

GESTATIONAL AND CHRONIC HYPERTENSION

If you develop gestational hypertension (which occurs after 20 weeks) or if you have had hypertension prior to pregnancy (chronic hypertension), you will need to be started on medications that are safe to take in pregnancy and that will prevent your blood pressure from going above 140/90. These medications may include *methyldopa*, *nifedipine*, or *labetalol*. Poorly controlled hypertension in pregnancy can lead to stroke or heart failure in the mother, poor growth of the fetus, or placental abruption. Once blood pressure is controlled during pregnancy, the outcome is often as successful as any other pregnancy. Delivery may occur before term if pressure cannot be controlled adequately. It is important to note, however, that these conditions increase the chances of having preeclampsia or eclampsia. Hypertension that persists after pregnancy is chronic hypertension and if not controlled can lead to additional long-term problems such as heart failure, renal failure, vision problems or loss of sight, or poor flow to vessels of the lower limbs.

C H A P T E R   1 2

OBESITY

OBESITY IS DEFINED as a body mass index (BMI) greater than thirty (determined by measuring your weight in kilograms divided by your height in metres squared; see page 18). A BMI greater than forty is considered morbid obesity. Obesity is the most common metabolic disorder of pregnancy. If you were previously obese and had bariatric surgery, it is important that your physician assesses you for any nutritional deficiencies. Some complications associated with obesity in pregnancy include first trimester miscarriage, preeclampsia and other hypertensive disorders, gestational diabetes, thromboembolic complications, and increased risk of malpresentation, large babies, late fetal loss, and increased fetal abnormalities, including neural tube defects.

It may be difficult for your physician to auscultate the fetal heart rate, or the lie and presentation of the fetus, at your antenatal visits if you are obese. An ultrasound late in the pregnancy may be needed to determine whether your baby is head first or lying in the correct position for vaginal delivery.

Complications in labour and postpartum include an increased risk of infection and an increase in preterm and postterm deliveries. It is harder to monitor the fetus in labour, and there is also an increased risk of failed induction (2.5 percent), slow progress in labour, epidural failure, birth trauma, high birth weight, fetal compromise, and the need for caesarean section.

Since obesity is associated with an increased risk of many complications in pregnancy, your physician may formulate a care plan that suggests some additional measures take place, such as recommending that you be seen by a dietician and the use of 5 mg folic acid (as opposed to 0.4 mg) to help prevent neural tube defects. Low-aerobic exercise may even be beneficial in pregnancy; however, weight loss is not desirable, but rather avoidance of excessive weight gain. It may be recommended that you be seen by the anaesthetist as there are increased anaesthetic risks associated with a high BMI as well. Moreover, *thromboembolism prophylaxis*, including the use of compression stockings (called *thromboembolic deterrent stockings*), in labour may be recommended, as there is an increased risk of clot in the legs and lungs. Some physicians may opt to even use an anticoagulant (such as *heparin*) for about seven days after delivery to further decrease the risk of blood clots (*venous thromboembolism*). There is also a risk of infection within the uterus after delivery in obese patients and also infection at the wound site if a caesarean section is done.

C H A P T E R 1 3

DIABETES

DIABETES IS A condition where there is an inability of the body to produce enough insulin or to respond to the insulin that is present to control the level of glucose in the blood. It occurs in about 6–9 percent of all pregnancies in the western world. The majority of these cases would have developed diabetes for the first time during pregnancy (called *gestational diabetes*). Gestational diabetes is diagnosed by performing a glucose test in either the first trimester or at 24 to 28 weeks. If this initial test is abnormal, another glucose test is done called an oral glucose tolerance test in which you will be given a special glucose drink and have a blood sample drawn just prior to the drink and one, two and three hours after. Elevated glucose levels in any two of the blood samples indicates the presence of gestational diabetes. Diabetes that is present prior to pregnancy is called *pregestational diabetes* and can be insulin dependent or type 1 (the body makes no natural insulin) or non–insulin dependent or type 2 (the body makes some insulin, but it is not used well).

Changes in the hormones in the body place a pregnant woman at greater risk of diabetes than a nonpregnant woman. Other things that increase your chances for diabetes are if you are over thirty-five years of age (over twenty-five in some populations); are obese; have diabetes in your family; are of Black, Asian, or Latino ethnicity; had gestational diabetes in a prior pregnancy and a previous baby that weighed more than 4000 g (about 8.5 lbs.); had a previous unexplained late fetal death; or are pregnant with multiples.

In the Caribbean particularly, the prevalence of diabetes is high, estimated at 11–18 percent among English-speaking regions.[4]

---

4 Michael S. Boyne, "Diabetes in the Caribbean: Trouble in Paradise," *Insulin* 4, no. 2 (2009): 94–105.

If diabetes is present prior to pregnancy, it is imperative that glucose is well controlled at least three months before conceiving to decrease risk to the fetus and to the mother during pregnancy. One of the main ways your glucose control is monitored is by checking your glucose levels daily at home and your doctor may also order a blood test called the HBA1c. When the HBA1c is less than 6.1 percent it can be presumed that glucose is controlled well. If the percentage is above this number, there is a high chance that you can have a baby with a congenital abnormality, a miscarriage, or a stillbirth. Certain medications that you may be taking prior to pregnancy may cause harm to the fetus, so all your medications should be reviewed with your obstetrician once you book for antenatal visits (or before conceiving if possible).

Your pregnancy may be managed by your obstetrician along with other physicians and healthcare specialists, such as an endocrinologist and dieticians, to ensure that there is the best outcome for you and your baby. There is a belief among some people that diabetes only pertains to sugar intake, but it is much more than that. The intake of total calories should be monitored, especially the amounts of carbohydrates, fats, and protein that are consumed. Low-impact exercises may change the way your body responds to insulin and improve glucose control. Frequency of antenatal visits will be increased. Tests will be done in the third trimester to assess how well the baby is doing and to monitor fetal growth (e.g., nonstress test and/or ultrasound).

Complications that can occur in pregnancy include preeclampsia, a large-for-gestational-age fetus, and stillbirths late in pregnancy. Additionally, those with pregestational diabetes may have worsening of eye disease, kidney disease, small babies (intrauterine growth restriction), and *diabetic ketoacidosis* (which is severely uncontrolled glucose levels that often require ICU admission to treat).

Medications used to treat diabetes will be based on the type of diabetes and the severity. Most commonly in pregnancy, insulin is considered the best option for attaining normal glucose levels. However, medications taken by mouth can be used, and these include *glyburide* or *metformin*. As the pregnancy advances, greater amounts of these medications may be needed. Your healthcare provider needs your assistance in achieving good glucose control, so you can partake in ensuring you keep a diary of your glucose levels at home and bring it to every antenatal visit. Glucose levels that are aimed for in pregnancy are as follows:

- Fasting levels ≤ 95 mg/dl
- Before meals ≤ 100 mg/dl
- 1 hour after meals ≤ 140 mg/dl
- 2 hours after meals ≤ 120 mg/dl
- HbA1c < 6.1 percent

Timing of delivery will be based on how well glucose was controlled throughout the pregnancy. Delivery may be before term (less than 37 weeks) if certain complications exist. Delivery is usually between 38 to 39 weeks gestation for diabetes that was monitored closely and very well controlled throughout pregnancy. If your baby is large (macrosomia) with an estimated fetal weight by ultrasound of greater than 4000 to 4500 grams (about 8.5 to 9.5 lbs.), a caesarean section may be done.

Babies born to diabetic mothers may have underdeveloped lungs and require a tube to be place in the air tube (trachea) to assist with breathing. They are also at risk of low blood glucose levels and admission to the neonatal intensive care unit.

C H A P T E R   1 4

ISSUES WITH THE UMBILICAL CORD AND PLACENTA

FUNCTIONS OF THE UMBILICAL CORD

THE UMBILICAL CORD connects a baby in the womb to its mother. It resembles a jump rope. It goes from an opening in your baby's abdomen (tummy) to the placenta, which is attached to the womb. The average cord is about 50 cm (20 inches) long.

In the placenta, oxygen and nutrients from your bloodstream pass into your baby's bloodstream and are carried to your baby along the umbilical cord. The umbilical cord inserts close to the centre of the placenta.

Blood circulates through vessels (circular tubes) in the cord, which is composed of one vein that carries blood rich in oxygen and nutrients from you to your baby, and two arteries that return oxygen-poor blood and waste products, such as carbon dioxide, from your baby back to the placenta. These blood vessels are wrapped in a gelatinous substance that insulates and protects them, called *Wharton's jelly*. This substance is also covered by a layer of membrane called the *amnion*.

POTENTIAL PROBLEMS WITH THE UMBILICAL CORD

TWO-VESSEL CORD

Occasionally (in 0.2–1 percent of pregnancies) the umbilical cord has only one artery (*single umbilical artery*), and the reason for this is not known. One artery can support an unborn baby through pregnancy and does not necessarily mean that there is a problem. However, it does increase the risk of the baby having problems that affect the heart, bones, intestines, or kidneys.

NUCHAL CORD

Movements of the baby can cause the umbilical cord to loop around the neck. There may be one or multiple loops. Think of being in a swimming pool with a lot of loose rope; inevitably you will swim through a loop at some point and it may hang over your neck. That is what happens in the uterus with the fetus. Similarly, the fetus may detangle from the loop just as readily. If cord is seen around your baby's neck during an ultrasound, do not be alarmed, a follow-up ultrasound may show that it is no longer there. Delivery can still be accomplished vaginally with a nuchal cord. However, during labour, abnormalities in fetal heart rate is possible. If this occurs and your baby is not coping well (determined by the CTG tracing and testing a fetal blood sample), your doctor may decide to perform a caesarean section.

TRUE KNOTS

These are very rare (1 percent) of pregnancies. Knots are most commonly seen in twin pregnancies where the babies share one amniotic sac (monoamniotic twin gestation) and in *polyhydramnios* (excessive amniotic fluid). As the baby moves about, the true knot forms. These knots are often not seen until delivery. They can increase the chance of a loss of the fetus in the antenatal period. Ultrasound cannot always detect this condition.

VASA PREVIA

This abnormality happens in one in twenty-five hundred pregnancies and is characterized when the fetal blood vessels travel uncovered (unprotected) through the amniotic membranes and cover or are too close to the cervix. It is associated with an abnormal insertion of the cord called *velamentous insertion*. This is when the umbilical cord inserts into the amniotic membranes instead of close to the centre of the placenta.

There are two types of vasa previa:

- Type I: the fetal vessels are in the amniotic membranes and overlie the cervix or are close to it.
- Type II: this happens if the placenta has more than one lobe and the vessels connecting the two lobes run over or are near the cervix.

This condition may be diagnosed on ultrasound. If you have this condition, your physician may coordinate your care with other specialists. Your provider may decide to give you a medication to help with fetal lung maturity and/or proceed with your delivery before your due date.

WHAT HAPPENS WITH THE CORD AFTER THE BABY IS BORN?

Soon after the birth, the person who performs the delivery will clamp the umbilical cord about 3–4 cm (1.5–2 inches) from your baby's belly button with a plastic clip then place another clamp at the other end of the cord, near the placenta. The cord will then be cut between the two clamps, leaving a stump about 2–3 cm (1–1.5 inches) long on your baby's belly button. Your healthcare provider will cut the cord, or with the provider's agreement, you or your birth partner could do it.

There are no nerves in the cord, so cutting it isn't painful for you or the baby. You can ask to have your baby lifted straight onto you before or right after the cord is cut if there are no complications at the time of delivery.

Between five and fifteen days after your baby is born, the umbilical stump will dry out, turn black, and drop off. Once the stump comes off, it usually takes about seven to ten days for the belly button to heal completely. Until the stump drops off and the belly button is completely healed, it's important to keep the area clean and dry to prevent infection. The stump should remain outside the diaper until it is healed.

Cord Blood

This is blood that is collected from your baby's umbilical cord and placenta right after delivery and it stored appropriately. Cord blood contains very young and important cells called *stem cells,* which can be used to treat certain diseases should your child develop them in future. Stem cells have the unique ability to transform themselves into many different types of cells. These cells are being used to treat many diseases, including sickle cell disease and cancers (such as leukemias and lymphomas). If this is something you may be interested in, discuss it with your doctor to see if there is an accredited cord blood bank in your area. These banks usually charge an annual storage fee after an initial payment.

FUNCTIONS OF THE PLACENTA

The placenta is a red and dusky blue tissue that is responsible for the transfer of oxygen to the fetus and waste products from the fetus back to the mother. It forms an intricate network of vessels and, as described earlier, is attached to the uterus of the mother and to the fetus via the umbilical cord (which is the conduit). The placenta is about 3 cm thick, 20 cm wide, and 400–600 grams by term. Once the baby is delivered, the placenta separates from the uterus within thirty minutes and is expelled out the vagina.

POTENTIAL PROBLEMS WITH THE PLACENTA

Placenta Previa

Placenta previa occurs when the placenta overlies the opening of the cervix or is close to it. It is divided into several types:

- *Low-lying:* The edge of the placenta is in the lower part of the uterus.
- *Marginal:* The placenta is within several centimetres away from the opening of the cervix.
- *Partial:* The placenta halfway covers the cervical opening.
- *Complete:* The placenta fully covers the cervical opening.

Placenta previa can cause bleeding anytime during pregnancy, but it is most common in the third trimester. If the bleeding is heavy and continued, your provider may have to deliver the baby before your due date. Sometimes the bleeding is light, occurs only for several days, and then stops. You must be carefully observed during your pregnancy if you have this condition. Your provider will often advise you to abstain from sexual intercourse, which can precipitate bleeding.

Women with low-lying and marginal placenta previa can sometimes be delivered vaginally. However, most often with partial and complete placenta previa, you must deliver by caesarean section to prevent death or extreme stress to the fetus that can lead to problems after birth, such as seizures or cerebral palsy. If you have placenta previa, you should have a full discussion with your provider so a decision can be made as to the best option for your delivery.

PLACENTAL ABRUPTION

This is when the placenta separates from the uterus before the baby is delivered. When this happens it opens up blood vessels in the uterus (at the point where the placenta was attached) and leads to bleeding. This blood can pass out through the vagina (*revealed abruption*) or be hidden and collect behind the placenta (*concealed abruption*).

Abruption is a serious emergency (in most cases), as it can cause the mother to bleed out her blood volume rapidly, and the fetus is also unable to receive its transfer of oxygen from the mother and can die. You are at an increased chance of having abruption if you had a threatened miscarriage in early pregnancy, smoke, use cocaine, have hypertension, are pregnant with multiples, have increased amniotic fluid around the baby (*polyhydramnios*), have placenta previa, incur infection within the amniotic sac (*chorioamnionitis*), have a blood-clotting disorder, sustain trauma to the abdomen (e.g., a car accident, a fall, or domestic violence), or have a procedure to turn the baby into the head-down position (*external cephalic version*).

If you experience any of the following symptoms, you may have an abruption and should go to the hospital immediately: vaginal bleeding with abdominal pain (which is usually continuous), contractions, abdomen is painful when touched, you feel like you will faint, or you do pass out. If bleeding is severe enough, it can lead to anemia and shock or death in the mother and fetal distress or death.

When you arrive at the hospital, if you are in labour and it is advanced (that is you will deliver within the next few minutes), you may be allowed to deliver vaginally. However, because of the risks to you and the baby are great, an emergency caesarean section may be required to deliver the baby and halt the bleeding.

If abruption occurs early in pregnancy and it is partial (i.e., only a small portion of the placenta separates), the bleeding stops, and the baby is not in any danger, your pregnancy may be allowed to progress until the baby's lungs are matured (usually around 32 to 34 weeks) and then you will be delivered.

ADHERENT PLACENTA

If the placenta does not detach within thirty minutes after the delivery, it is called a *retained placenta*. One of the reasons it may not separate is because of a condition where the placenta is abnormally attached to the uterus. This condition can cause severe postpartum haemorrhage, and if bleeding is uncontrollable may cause your physician to have to make the decision to remove your entire uterus in order to save your life because of continued bleeding.

This condition is rare, occurring in only about one in twenty-five hundred pregnancies. Conditions that increase the chances of having an adherent placenta include a previous caesarean section, previous surgery to remove uterine fibroids, and placenta previa.

There are three types of adherent placentas:

1. *Accreta*: the placenta is attached to the muscle of the uterus instead of only the surface layer of the uterus. This placenta can be separated, but with difficulty.
2. *Increta*: the placenta goes into the muscle fibers of the uterus.
3. *Percreta*: the placenta goes through the muscle fiber to the outside of the uterus and attaches to other organs around it (e.g., the bladder or bowel).

This condition may sometimes be seen during the antenatal period during an ultrasound. In this case, your healthcare provider may plan a caesarean section with other experts to aim for the best outcome for you and your baby.

Accessory Placental Lobes

This is when there is an extra lobe of placenta a little distance away from the main placenta. It can cause problems after delivery as it may be retained after the main placental is delivered and lead to postpartum haemorrhage or infection if it is not detected and removed.

Tumors in the Placenta

The placenta can have tumors (extra tissue growths) made up of blood vessels that can cause bleeding in pregnancy or even death of the fetus. However, these tumors are extremely rare.

CHAPTER 15

VACCINATIONS

DURING PRENATAL CARE, your healthcare provider will ensure that your vaccinations are up to date. Vaccines that are generally safe for a mother to receive during pregnancy include diphtheria, tetanus, pertussis, influenza, and hepatitis B vaccine. Tetanus, diphtheria, and pertussis (Tdap) vaccine is routinely given between 27 and 36 weeks gestation to protect your newborn against pertussis (whooping cough) until he or she gets the DTaP vaccine at two months of age. If Tdap is given early in pregnancy, it does not need to be given again at 27–36 weeks. Some vaccines may not have outright evidence that they are harmful in pregnancy; however, they have not been studied enough in the setting of pregnancy and therefore they should not be given in pregnancy. These include measles, mumps, rubella, varicella, and BCG (a vaccine against tuberculosis). Some vaccines have to be considered on a case-by-case basis.

ANTHRAX

When the risk for exposure to aerosolized (particles carried in the air) *Bacillus anthracis* spores is low, vaccination of pregnant women is not recommended. When there is a high risk for exposure to aerosolized *B. anthracis* spores, pregnancy is neither a precaution nor a contraindication to post-exposure prophylaxis (PEP). Pregnant women at risk for inhalation anthrax should receive AVA (which is the name of the anthrax vaccine) and sixty days of treatment.

JAPANESE ENCEPHALITIS

Japanese encephalitis is the leading cause of viral encephalitis in Asian countries. A vaccine against it is recommended for those with significant risk of exposure.

TYPHOID

Neither form of the typhoid vaccine is recommended in pregnancy.

POLIO

Polio is an enterovirus with three different strains. The inactivated polio vaccine (IPV) should be avoided if possible but used if you are at an increased risk of infection and require immediate protection against polio.

PNEUMOCOCCAL

There are currently two pneumococcal vaccines available for use:

1. *Pneumococcal Conjugate (PCV13)* does not have pregnancy recommendations at this time, and its use is limited among women of childbearing age.
2. *Pneumococcal Polysaccharide (PPSV23)* use during the first trimester of pregnancy has not been evaluated for safety; however, no adverse consequences have been reported among newborns whose mothers were unintentionally vaccinated during pregnancy. This vaccine can be given during pregnancy. It is particularly important that women with conditions such as sickle cell disease receive this vaccine.

CHOLERA

Cholera is an acute diarrheal disease. This vaccine is not recommended in pregnancy.

PLAGUE

Plague is a disease caused by *Yersinia pestis*. It is transmitted if a human is bitten by an infected rat or flea. However, the vaccine is not recommended for pregnant patients.

HEPATITIS A

This vaccine is produced from inactivated virus (meaning the harmful components of the hepatitis A have been destroyed chemically); therefore, the risk to the developing fetus is low. So if you are travelling to an area that has a high risk of exposure to hepatitis A, the risks compared to the benefits should be discussed with your healthcare provider. If you are exposed, immune globulin is strongly recommended.

RABIES

Because of the potential consequences of inadequately managed rabies exposure, pregnancy is not considered a contraindication to PEP. Some studies have indicated no increased incidence of abortion, premature births, or fetal abnormalities associated with rabies vaccination. If the risk of exposure to rabies is substantial, PEP also might be indicated during pregnancy. Rabies exposure or the diagnosis of rabies in the mother should not be regarded as reasons to terminate the pregnancy.

VACCINIA (SMALLPOX)

Smallpox vaccine should not be administered in a pre-event setting to pregnant women, women who are trying to become pregnant, or women who intend to become pregnant in the following four weeks.

Smallpox vaccination during pregnancy should not ordinarily be a reason to terminate pregnancy. Pregnant women who have had a definite exposure to smallpox virus (i.e., face-to-face, household, or close-proximity contact with a smallpox patient) and are, therefore, at high risk for contracting the disease should be vaccinated. Smallpox infection among pregnant women has been reported to result in a more severe infection than among nonpregnant women.

YELLOW FEVER

Pregnancy is a precaution for yellow fever vaccine administration compared with most other live vaccines (in which the harmful components have been lessened), which are contraindicated in pregnancy. If travel is unavoidable, and the risks for yellow fever exposure are felt to outweigh the vaccination risks, a pregnant woman should be vaccinated. However, inadvertent vaccination is not a cause for termination.

INFLUENZA

The inactivated form if the influenza vaccine may be given during pregnancy either during or before the influenza season.

RUBELLA

Also known as German measles. Tests for the antibodies to rubella are routinely done in pregnancy. If this test is positive it means you are immune to rubella. Tests that are negative or levels are low suggest you are not immune. The vaccination, however, cannot be given during pregnancy, only after delivery to protect future pregnancies. An acute rubella infection in a nonimmunized woman can be detrimental to the baby, causing abnormalities that may lead to fetal death or that may be incompatible with life outside the womb.

CHAPTER 16

NERVOUS SYSTEM DISORDERS

EPILEPSY

A seizure is due to abnormal activity in the nerve cells of the brain, and some women have a seizure disorder called epilepsy. This is the most common nerve disorder to complicate pregnancy and may be classified into different types depending on the type of seizure that is experienced. Most cases of epilepsy have no underlying cause; in some it may be a result of surgeries, lesions in the brain, or *antiphospholipid syndrome*.

Epilepsy has some implications for your pregnancy. The frequency of your seizures may increase or decrease. The seizures may also increase after the delivery of the baby. If you are on medications, you should consult with your provider to determine if it is appropriate for you to change medication or your dose. You will also be required to take 4 mg of folic acid instead of the usual 0.4 mg required during pregnancy. It is important to remember that if you are well and seizure-free, your fetus will do well. Ensure that you stay calm and get adequate rest during the pregnancy and the labour process.

It is important to understand that you may have increased risk of some complications, however, such as preterm labour, preeclampsia, and congenital abnormalities such as neural tube defects, heart defects, and facial defects. Seizures can cause your water to break or cause placental abruption (especially if you have several sequentially).

Seek the care of your healthcare provider before pregnancy to decrease the risks. Your infant may also have an increased risk of seizure disorder. In most cases your medication should not interfere with your ability to breastfeed.

MIGRAINES

Migraines are common in pregnancy. They may appear for the first time in pregnancy (especially the third trimester) or worsen in previously diagnosed sufferers. It may present as a throbbing unilateral headache. A person may have symptoms that precede it as well, such as sensitivity to light, sensitivity to noise, nausea, and vomiting. Some medications may be used, such as beta-blockers, aspirin, and other medications.

MULTIPLE SCLEROSIS

In this disorder there are multiple sites that are demyelinated in the brain and the spinal cord. This means that the protective sheath (myelin) that covers the nerve fibres is damaged. If you have *neuropathic bladder* as a result of your multiple sclerosis (MS), you may have increased problems with urinary tract infections during pregnancy, otherwise there is no long-term effect on pregnancy and breastfeeding. You may have fewer attacks of MS while pregnant and more in the postpartum period.

MYASTHENIA GRAVIS

In this disorder there are antibodies produced by your body that affect the *nicotinic acetylcholine receptor* on the motor end plates of your muscle fibres. This interferes with nerve transmission, and as a result you may experience muscle weakness and fatigue. For women who are pregnant with this illness, it may get worse, get better, or stay the same.

If you have this disorder, it is important to see your healthcare provider. Additional monitoring may be required for the fetus, as there is an increased chance of issues with the growth of your fetus, early labour, and a disorder where the fetus may develop limb contractures in the womb called *arthrogryposis multiplex congenita*. You may find that the first stage of labour may occur without any difficulty, but the second part may be very hard. Allowing a vaginal delivery is preferable, but it will be important for your anaesthesiologist and obstetrician to formulate a delivery plan.

BELL'S PALSY

Most cases of Bell's palsy are caused by a latent herpes simplex virus type I infection. In pregnancy the cause may be due to a swelling of the nerve in the temporal bone. The diagnosis is a clinical one. You may experience facial weakness of the frontal muscle resulting in the inability to wrinkle your face on the affected side. You may have pain in the ear on that side and a loss of taste. The symptoms may occur close to your due date or shortly after delivery. Most times Bell's palsy gets better on its own, but sometimes medication may be required. Please see you doctor immediately if you have any of the above symptoms.

CARPAL TUNNEL SYNDROME

When the median nerve of the arm is compressed due to the retention of fluid that occurs during pregnancy, you may experience tingling and numbness in your thumb and two lateral fingers. You may have an increase in symptoms at night that may be relieved if the wrist is massaged or moved. This will most likely improve after delivery. You may also use wrist splints to support the wrist and avoid flexion. Additional medical or surgical management may be warranted in severe cases.

OTHER NERVE COMPLICATIONS

Other nerve complications may include *meralgia paraesthetica*, which is pain on the front of the thigh that is a result of nerve compression, or *foot drop*. The former may happen if you are overweight, and it usually improves after delivery. The latter may occur if there is damage to the sciatic nerve as a result of a prolonged second stage of labour or if there is a large fetus putting pressure on your lower back compressing the nerve.

C H A P T E R   1 7

SKIN DISORDERS

THE SKIN CHANGES in pregnancy, such a stretch marks and darkening of the pigment of the skin (*melasma*), are due to hormonal effects. When darkening occurs around the nose and on the cheeks, it is called *chloasma*. In most women there is a darkening of a line that runs down the middle of your tummy, from the hair line of the genitals to the belly button, called a *linea nigra*.

ECZEMA AND ATOPIC ECZEMA

Eczema is the most common skin disorder of pregnancy. Some of you may have eczema before pregnancy and it tends to worsen in pregnancy in about half of those afflicted, but many cases develop in the second and third trimesters of pregnancy. This skin disorder does not affect the pregnancy; however, it may affect maternal comfort levels. It may be important for you to consult with your skin doctor and obstetrician to find the best treatment plan. Skin emollients may provide useful. However, if your case is severe, topical steroids may be warranted under the guidance of a healthcare professional.

POLYMORPHIC ERUPTION OF PREGNANCY

Also known as *prurigo of pregnancy* or *pruritic urticarial papules and plaques of pregnancy*, this is the second most common skin condition in pregnancy happening in the third trimester or postpartum. You may have itchy red plaques (which are slighted raise areas of the skin) and papules (which are like tiny little bump or vesicles). The outbreak usually starts on the stomach around the

137

areas of the stretch marks but skips the belly button area. It may look patchy, like a world map with the outbreak representing landmasses. It may include the arms, thighs, breasts, and buttocks. It skips the face, soles of feet, and palms of the hands. The condition goes away close to term or shortly after delivery, and it is not known to have any a negative impact on the outcome of pregnancy.

PRURITIC FOLLICULITIS OF PREGNANCY

An acne-like breakout that occurs on the shoulders, upper back of arms, chest, and abdomen.

PEMPHIGOID GESTATIONIS

Pemphigoid gestationis is an autoimmune condition (which means the body is attacking itself) that usually starts in the second or third trimester. It starts in the belly button area, and the skin lesions are itchy, red initially, with areas of blisters. This skin disorder may improve towards the end of pregnancy but may recur again after delivery. The baby may have similar lesions, and there may be some risks to the infant.

INTRAHEPATIC CHOLESTASIS OF PREGNANCY

This condition is linked to itching without a rash in the first or last part of pregnancy. The itching is cause by high bile levels in the mother's blood. Bile is a greenish fluid produced in the liver and stored in the gallbladder that helps in the digestion of food. The itchiness may cause you to scratch, causing stretch marks on arms, legs, back, and abdomen. Itching usually starts on the palms of hands and soles of feet. Medications can be used to decrease bile levels.

This skin condition can have a significant impact on your pregnancy by increasing the risk of problems with the baby, such as early deliver, meconium passage within the uterus (baby's first stool which could be aspirated into the lungs), and death of the baby in the uterus. As the mom, you may have problems with blood clotting. You have a high chance of this condition happening in a future pregnancy if you have had it before. You may also have an increased chance of having gallstones in the future.

C H A P T E R   1 8

CANCER

CANCER IS AN uncontrolled overgrowth of cells within the body that invades surrounding tissue and can spread to other places in the body. There are many different things that may cause one person to develop cancer over another. Some of these factors include a history of cancer in the family, certain chemicals in the environment, sexually transmitted viruses, obesity, and ethnicity.

A diagnosis of cancer can be overwhelming for both the pregnant mother and her family. If you have been diagnosed with cancer there may be many questions in your mind, including will I be able to carry this pregnancy to term or will cancer be transmitted to my baby? Can I be treated while I am pregnant? What about breastfeeding? We will answer these questions for you.

Cancer is not common in pregnancy, occurring in about one in every one thousand to fifteen hundred pregnancies. Its diagnosis can be delayed or even missed because symptoms of cancer can be similar to symptoms of pregnancy described earlier. Cancer in the skin is commonly seen; however, in the Caribbean, the larger percentage of ethnicities of darker skin tones makes it a little less common in this region. Any type of cancer can be encountered in pregnancy; however, the types seen in women during the years they can become pregnant are cervical, breast, ovarian, leukemia, lymphomas, thyroid, and bowel cancer. How to treat each type of cancer in pregnancy is beyond the scope of this book; however, there are general principles in how to approach women who do have cancer. You and your healthcare providers (an obstetrician and cancer specialist) must come up with a plan that is specific for your case and stage of the disease. Some of the treatment used can cause loss of the fetus or harmful effects when used in the first and second trimester, therefore a decision to use some form of treatment must be made on an individual basis.

There are several options for treatment of cancer in pregnancy (other than surgery). Surgery may be used in combination with these methods. As noted in the first section of this book, major development of organs occur in the first trimester, therefore use of these cancer treatment below can cause miscarriage or abnormalities in organs when used in the first trimester.

1. *Chemotherapy*: This is the use of drugs used to slow or stop the growth of cancer cells. There are drugs that are safe to use in the second and third trimester. Effects to the fetus are very small but may include a small baby, premature delivery, and (rarely) stillbirths. Chemotherapy is not used three weeks before delivery, as it can affect the baby from producing adequate blood cells, which can lead to anemia, infection, or bleeding.

2. *Radiotherapy:* This uses ionizing radiation to kill cancer cells. It can be directed to a specific site in the body or given to the whole body. It can be used after 16 weeks of pregnancy only, but not near the uterus with the baby. This can lead to the possibility of cancer in the fetus (e.g., leukemias and lymphomas) manifesting in childhood or later in life.

<u>CERVICAL CANCER</u>

This is the most frequent cancer (relating to women only) occurring in pregnancy. Pap smear screening is a routine test done in pregnancy (for the reason stated in section 1); there are those infrequent times, however, that it identifies cervical cancer. Pregnancy does not worsen the cancer, and no cancer cells are transferred to the fetus.

Very early stage disease can be treated in the second trimester by removing the portion of the cervix affected by the disease. This is called *cold knife cone biopsy*. There is still a chance to have bleeding, infection, and loss of the pregnancy with this treatment.

Later stages are treated by radiotherapy by high doses. In the first or early second trimester, consequently, there will be spontaneous loss of the fetus because of the radiation. If the pregnancy is not miscarried, there will be abnormalities in the fetus. In this late stage and period of pregnancy, some physicians may offer you complete removal of the womb (hysterectomy), which would result in loss of the fetus and the ability to become pregnant again.

Patients that are diagnosed in the late second or third trimester usually can receive corticosteroids to assist in maturing the baby's lungs, and then the baby is delivered by caesarean section. The reason a C-section is required is because the spread of the disease can cause the cervix to tear and bleed uncontrollably during vaginal delivery, and this can even cause widespread infection in the mother.

BREAST CANCER

This occurs in about one in three thousand pregnancies. Pregnancy does not worsen breast cancer and treatment is the same as if it was a nonpregnant female. In certain regions of the Caribbean, there is a high occurrence of breast cancer. In fact, a study has shown that the Bahamas has the highest number of breast cancer gene abnormalities than anywhere in the world.[5]

Cancerous breast tumours tend to be larger and more advanced in stage when they are discovered; this happens because lumps felt are often thought to be a result of breast milk production (which is the most common cause of a breast lump in pregnancy). If a lump is found in pregnancy, you may need a mammogram and a biopsy to diagnosis it.

Treatment would include surgery to remove the lump or the entire breast(s) affected. If just the lump is removed, radiotherapy is usually also needed and is safe in early pregnancy, but in late pregnancy it can still expose the fetus (even when a shield is used over the abdomen to block the radiation). As stated

---

5 Talia Donenberg, John Lunn, DuVaughn Curling, Theodore Turnquest, Elisa Krill-Jackson, Robert Royer, Steven A. Narod, and Judith Hurley, "A High Prevalence of BRCA1 Mutations among Breast Cancer Patients from the Bahamas," *Breast Cancer Research and Treatment (2011)* 125 (2): 591–96.

earlier, chemotherapy is safe in pregnancy and is often used in the second and third trimester before or after surgery.

CAN I BREASTFEED IF I HAVE BREAST CANCER?

Cancer cells are not transferred into breast milk; therefore breastfeeding is safe. An exception to this is if you are receiving chemotherapy or a drug called *tamoxifen*, as they can pass into breast milk and are harmful to the nursing neonate. If breast surgery was recent, it may be best not to breastfeed; the surgeon performing the surgery will advise you appropriately. The tumour or surgery on the breast can affect the system of tubes (ducts) that carry and produce breast milk, resulting in a decrease in milk. If you notice breast milk supply is low, you will have to supplement feeding with infant formula. It is important that you consult your paediatrician on issues with breastfeeding and the need for supplementation.

CAN I HAVE ANOTHER BABY AFTER BEING TREATED FOR BREAST CANCER?

Breast cancer in some cases is curable. It is, however, suggested by most obstetric authorities that it is best to wait two years after breast cancer treatment before attempting pregnancy. When pregnancy occurs sooner than this, it can lead to recurrence of the cancer.

OVARIAN CANCER

This is not a very common cancer. However, it is ranked the deadliest cancer of the female reproductive organs.

Ovarian masses can be found in pregnancy and most often these are *cysts* (which are like fluid-filled balloons that can be small or large). In early pregnancy these noncancerous cysts help to produce hormones to maintain the pregnancy, and they go away by the second trimester.

There are usually no symptoms of ovarian cancer, but when a cyst is seen on the ultrasound, it can be observed by repeating the scan several weeks apart to determine if it is growing or changing. The way an ovarian mass looks on an ultrasound may cause the healthcare provider to suspect ovarian cancer. The mass would have to be removed to confirm if it is cancer. This surgery will remove the mass, the ovary, and the tube on the affected side and is safe in pregnancy. Chemotherapy can also be used in combination with surgery. After delivery, more extensive treatment may be required depending on the stage of the disease.

CHAPTER 19

SICKLE CELL DISEASE

SICKLE CELL DISEASE is the most common inherited condition worldwide. It is a group of inherited single gene autosomal recessive disorders that result in a change in the shape of the red blood cell. As a result, these cells are fragile and break down easier than non-sickle-shaped cells. They also may get trapped in blood vessels. This causes an anemia and blockage of small blood vessels. Other issues include stroke, pulmonary hypertension (high pressure in the vessels of the lungs), leg ulcers, kidney disease, eye disease, gallbladder disease, and bone disease of the hip.

Sickle cell disease is common in people of African and Indian descent. These ethnicities make up a large proportion of the population within the Caribbean region. In fact, there are sickle-cell clinics devoted to only these patients in several Caribbean countries (including the Bahamas and Jamaica).

Pregnancy if you have sickle cell may have some increased risks that may affect you and the pregnancy. Some of these include an increased rate of fetal loss due to spontaneous abortion. With this in mind, if you are considering pregnancy, you should see your healthcare provider for preconceptual counselling and have your vaccines brought up to date. Also, certain medications used in sickle cell disease (e.g., *hydroxyurea*) should not be used while trying to conceive or during the first trimester of pregnancy.

It may be useful to have the father screened to know his *haemoglobinopathy status* (whether he has sickle cell disease or the trait) as well. The trait means that only a part of the gene is being carried. Here are some possibilities of your baby having sickle cell. If you have the disease and:

- the father has the trait, there is a 50 percent chance the baby will have sickle cell disease.
- the father has sickle cell disease, there is a 100 percent chance that the baby will have the disease.
- the father does not have the trait or disease, there is a 100 percent chance that the baby will have the trait.

If both parents have the trait, the baby has 25 percent of having the sickle cell disease.

Your provider may consider starting you on medication to reduce the risk of preeclampsia (high blood pressure in pregnancy). Iron supplementation may be recommended if there is evidence of iron deficiency. They may also give you medication to prevent clots if you are admitted to the hospital.

Painful *sickle cell crisis* is one of the most common complications during pregnancy and the most common cause of admission to the hospital. This involves pain in the limbs, back, and sometimes chest and abdomen. Crises can increase in pregnancy or remain at the same frequency as when you were not pregnant. If you are having symptoms of pain, you should contact your healthcare provider.

Placenta previa and abruption occur due to hypoxia (lack of oxygen) and placental infarction. Preterm (early) labour is another possible complication. Growth of the baby may be monitored on regular intervals with the use of ultrasound. If you have any vaginal bleeding or abdominal pain let your provider know.

With these complications in mind, it is important that you meet with your healthcare provider prior to conception, continue your folic acid at 5 mg once a day, keep hydrated during the course of pregnancy, and seek help early in the event of a crisis or if you are feeling unwell.

You may require a review with the anaesthesiologist to plan the best analgesia anaesthesia for your delivery. Planning ahead is a good idea to achieve the best outcome for your pregnancy.

C H A P T E R   2 0

MENTAL HEALTH

PREGNANCY IS A life altering occurrence that comes with many changes—such as changes in your body, relationships, work role, home role—as well as fear of pregnancy outcomes and delivery. If you have had mental health challenges in the past, it currently increases your risk of issues with this area during pregnancy. Be sure to discuss your pregnancy plans with your mental health provider.

"You keep him in perfect peace whose mind is stayed on you,
because he trusts in you."

— ISAIAH 26:3 (ESV)

BABY BLUES

This is a time when you may feel tearful or sad with no explainable reason. You may be moody or sensitive to the response of others, have a loss of appetite, not sleep well, be unable to concentrate well, and have a loss of interest or pleasure in doing things. These symptoms are thought to be due to the hormonal changes taking place in the body during and just after delivery. A new baby in the house causes adjustments in the routine and can be a significant factor in the development or increase of the baby blues.

The baby blues normally resolves within days. Support is the most beneficial component in dealing with this. However, if this does not improve then you must consider seeking help from a healthcare provider.

POSTPARTUM DEPRESSION

Depression symptoms include feeling unhappy or tearful, irritable, and/or tired and unable to sleep as well as changes in appetite, loss of hope, negative or guilty thoughts, and suicidal thoughts. Depression during the antenatal period puts you at increased risk for depression in the postpartum period. Other risk factors for depression include:

- Substance abuse
- Previous episodes of depression
- A family history of depression
- A lack of support
- Being unhappy about the pregnancy
- Negative life events with yourself or partner

Depression symptoms last longer and may be more intense than the baby blues. These symptoms last at least two weeks. It may be difficult to carry out daily activities. Symptoms may start during pregnancy or shortly thereafter.

Many times postpartum depression is observed in the mother, but it can also occur in the father as well. It is important to pay attention to the father and his reaction during pregnancy and thereafter.

PSYCHOSIS

Psychosis, although uncommon, can be life-threatening to yourself, your infant, and your family. Its onset is sudden with severe symptoms within two to three weeks of delivery. It is important to be aware of the warning signs:

- Confusion of your mind (you may start to imagine things)
- Behaviours that appear to be a break with reality (inappropriate behaviour)
- Mood swings
- Inability to sleep
- Restless, agitated behaviours

If you have had a previous episode of psychosis or bipolar disorder, you are at an increased risk of it occurring again during the postpartum (or pregnancy) period. Urgent medical attention is needed to ensure your safety and the safety of those that are around you.

BIPOLAR DISORDER AND SCHIZOPHRENIA

The information of these illnesses in pregnancy is limited. Some ladies improve during pregnancy while others may worsen or stay the same. The course during and after pregnancy is influenced by the number and severity of previous episodes, quality of support systems, and understanding the disease process.

EATING DISORDERS

Anorexia nervosa and *bulimia nervosa* are eating disorders that can have serious effects in pregnancy. Women with anorexia nervosa starve themselves until they are severely underweight because they feel they are fat or do not want to become fat. In extreme cases women starve themselves to death. Women with bulimia eat large amounts of food, but then force themselves to vomit afterwards; some even take laxatives to cause loose stools. If you have a current eating disorder, this may increase your risk of miscarriage, decrease birth weight in the infant, increase chances of hyperemesis gravidarum or gestational diabetes, increase the need for caesarean section, and increase the chances of postpartum depression. Eating disorders may improve during pregnancy.

ANXIETY AND ANXIETY DISORDERS

As stated earlier, pregnancy is a time with lots of changes in your body and your mind. It may be uncharted territory if this is your first pregnancy or murky seas if you had a previous bad experience. To have concerns and fears is not an uncommon occurrence. So do not feel that you are the only one if you are experiencing anxiety or that you have to brave it alone. When anxiety symptoms evolve to anxiety attacks or panic attacks, it is an anxiety disorder. Pay attention to the following symptoms of anxiety:

- Feeling irritable and overwhelmed
- Feeling overanxious all the time and not able to control it
- Worrying about events and activities, such a constant worry about your baby
- Being unable to concentrate, mind going blank
- Inability to sleep (insomnia)
- Tense muscles causing neck and back pain

Anyone can develop anxiety, but there are some things that make it more likely:

- If you have family members that have anxiety or panic attacks
- If you have had anxiety or panic attacks in the past
- If you have experienced a traumatic event
- If you are using drugs
- If you have depression
- If you are under extra stress

Anxiety poses risks for moms, such as increased risk for postpartum depression and postpartum anxiety. Women with anxiety have more physical ailments during pregnancy and may be at risk for post–traumatic stress symptoms after childbirth.

Some research has found that babies of anxious mothers may be susceptible to preterm birth. There's also evidence that the mom's anxiety may affect her infant's and lead to behavioural and emotional issues in childhood. The good news is that anxiety during pregnancy is treatable, and there are some things that you can do to cope with anxiety and cut down on your anxiety at work and at home:

- Incorporate regular exercise such as swimming, walking, deep breathing exercises, or stretching into your routine.

- Eat a healthy, well-balanced diet. Incorporate omega-3 fatty acids found in fish and seafood to reduce depression.
- Do not stay up late. Go to bed at a timely hour.
- Reduce your chores and find time for relaxation options such as a nap, reading a book, or doing a favorite hobby.
- Say no. You can't do everything by yourself. Consider slowing down a priority, and ask your friends and loved ones for help as needed. Decline extra projects or tasks.
- Adjust your work schedule. Take advantage of vacation time.
- Reduce your commute. Consider adjusting your work hours to avoid the traffic, consider taking public transportation, carpooling, or getting dropped at work.
- Monitor the information you are exposing yourself to. Reading pregnancy books (such as this one!) and surfing pregnancy websites for information is good, but remember the many complications that are discussed probably will not happen during your pregnancy. Focus on positive thoughts and a positive outcome.
- Join (or create!) a support group. If you're coping with a difficult situation, connecting with other moms-to-be dealing with similar issues may be helpful.
- Review your finances; make a list of things that you will need for the new addition and purchase them one item at a time over time or borrow them from a friend or family member. People love to chip in when a new baby is on the way.
- Prepare for family life; parenting is something you learn along the way. If you have any friends with young babies, plan to spend time with them. Allow the Holy Spirit to lead you in training up your child properly.
- Spend time praying, reading your Bible, and meditating on the Word of God.

Be aware that healthcare providers may not regularly screen for anxiety. Hence, if you are struggling with anxiety or anxious thoughts, it's very important to talk to your obstetrician, talk to your partner, and talk to a family member or spiritual leader. If your healthcare provider doesn't appear to be knowledgeable about anxiety disorders or dismisses your concerns, find another for a proper diagnosis and treatment. For instance, you might make an appointment with a mental health professional or a psychiatrist.

If you have been diagnosed with an anxiety disorder, then psychological therapies mentioned earlier can be used. However, more study is needed on its use in pregnant women. Antidepressants—specifically *selective serotonin reuptake inhibitors* (SSRIs) and *benzodiazepines*—are commonly prescribed for anxiety disorders and have been shown to reduce symptoms. However, there are risks associated with these medications.

Getting help during pregnancy will protect you and your baby from unnecessary risks and reduce your chances of postpartum anxiety and depression.

> *"Be anxious for nothing, but in everything by prayer and supplication, with thanksgiving, let your requests be made known to God; and the peace of God, which surpasses all understanding, will guard your hearts and minds through Christ Jesus."*
>
> —PHILIPPIANS 4:6–7 (NKJV)

It is thought that 5–16 percent of women struggle with an anxiety disorder during pregnancy or postpartum. These disorders include:

- *Obsessive-compulsive disorder,* in which there are repetitive and often distressing, anxious thoughts that cannot be controlled and lead to repetitive actions (e.g., washing the hands or body from dirt, checking to see if the doors are locked, and collecting, or hoarding items with no obvious value.)
- *Panic disorders* that include attacks where there is a sudden feeling of fear that is out of proportion to the true situation. Symptoms may

include a racing heart, fear of impending death, sweating, chest pain, and difficulty breathing.
- *Phobias* or intense fears of objects or situations, such as flying, heights, closed-in spaces, and animals.

These anxiety disorders can easily cause a pregnant woman to avoid leaving home and coming for antenatal care and, in turn, place her and her baby at risk for bad outcomes during or after delivery.

TREATMENT FOR MENTAL ILLNESSES
MEDICATIONS
If you are on medication, please do not stop it suddenly unless instructed by your physician as this may cause a relapse of your condition or side effects.

PSYCHOLOGICAL THERAPIES
These therapies help people to change the way they think about themselves and the world by changing negative thoughts to positive ones.

> *"And now dear brothers and sisters, one final thing. Fix your thoughts on what is true, and honorable, and right, and pure, and lovely, and admirable. Think about things that are excellent and worthy of praise."*

> —PHILIPPIANS 4:8 (NLT)

Other therapies aim to improve communication skills between the mother and persons whom she interacts with (e.g., family, friends, coworkers, etc.).

> *"If it be possible, as much as lieth in you, live peaceably with all men."*

> —ROMANS 12:18 (KJV)

These methods may prove beneficial and may assist or be used in place of medications depending on the mental health illness. A discussion with a mental health provider will help determine which treatment suits your needs.

"Why am I discouraged? Why is my heart so sad? I will put my hope in God! I will praise Him again—my Savior and my God!"

—Psalm 42:11 (NLT)

CHAPTER 21

HYPEREMESIS GRAVIDARUM

VOMITING IS QUITE common in pregnancy; up to 70 percent of women experience it. However, vomiting in pregnancy that is severe enough to cause dehydration, weight loss, and changes in the electrolytes in the body is known as *hyperemesis gravidarum*. This only affects 0.5 percent to 2 percent of pregnancies. The hormone hCG is the main contributing factor to this condition. When its level reaches its highest, which is around 10 weeks, is when the condition tends to be at its worse. Symptoms tend to begin at 5 to 6 weeks gestation and resolve by 16 weeks. Women that are pregnant with multiples (twins or greater), have a thyroid disease, or have an abnormal type of pregnancy known as a *molar pregnancy* are more susceptible to this condition.

If you have persistent vomiting or are unable to keep down any food or drink, contact your healthcare provider. Hyperemesis gravidarum may cause you to have to be admitted to the hospital to get fluids intravenously and medications to decrease nausea and vomiting. Some of these medications include *dimenhydrinate* (Gravol®), *promethazine* (Phenergan®), vitamin B12, and vitamin B6 in combination with *doxylamine* (Diclectin®).

If you have vomiting in pregnancy, changing the food you eat may help. Avoid spicy food or odors that may upset your stomach. Even food that tastes good may be one that upsets your stomach.

Eat snacks between small meals to prevent your stomach from getting empty. Snack on food and meals that are easy to digest, such as the BRATT diet (banana, rice, applesauce, toast, and tea). Ginger teas, mints, and even tablets may be helpful for a queasy stomach.

Pregnancy does not mean that you must eat the portion size of two; although you must maintain a healthy diet, do not overeat as this, too, can contribute to vomiting in a person with hyperemesis gravidarum in pregnancy.

"Beloved, I pray that all may go well with you and that you may be in good health, as it goes well with your soul."

—3 JOHN 1:2 (ESV)

CHAPTER 22

HIV AND OTHER SEXUALLY TRANSMITTED INFECTIONS

SEXUALLY TRANSMITTED INFECTIONS are infections that are transmitted most commonly through sexual contact, although some (e.g., HIV) can be transmitted in other ways. Sexual contact includes vaginal intercourse or intercourse in the back passage, contact of the penis or vagina with the mouth, and in some instances genital skin-to-skin contact without penetration of the penis. It is important that tracing and treatment of person(s) with whom you are sexually active with be done. If curable infections are not treated, reinfection will occur.

There are situation in which STIs are contracted that are out of a person's control including; sexual abuse, congenital infections and exposure to blood products or it can be a consequence of decisions made without knowing all the risks like intravenous drug use. It is God's desire that we be free from diseases, including sexually transmitted infections. Here we will discuss some of the more common infections that are encountered in pregnancy.

HUMAN IMMUNODEFICIENCY VIRUS (HIV)

HIV is a virus that infects cells in the body that normally fight off infection (the immune cells). The virus eventually destroys these cells, making one defenseless to other infections that can cause severe illness or death.

HIV is a common infection in women of childbearing age. All women are tested for HIV infection when they book for antenatal care. This is to identify those mothers that are infected to prevent mother-to-child transmission.

Mother-to-child transmission can occur during pregnancy, delivery as the baby passes through the birth canal (*vertical transmission*), or through breastfeeding. HIV is transmitted by sexual contact, needle sticks (as in drug users sharing needles), and by blood transfusion with infected blood (less commonly).

A person can have HIV for years before showing any symptoms. When symptoms appear, it is when the immune cells fall to a low level and infections occur, at this point the person has AIDS (*acquired immune deficiency syndrome*).

If you are positive for HIV or test positive for the first time during pregnancy, many questions may arise in your mind.

WILL MY BABY GET HIV FROM ME?

Not necessarily! The use of medications called *antiretrovirals* have significantly decreased the chances of babies being infected from a mother to less than 2 percent. This includes the use of three types of HIV drugs used in combination that lower the level of the virus in the blood. It is extremely important that you take your medication every day in order for it to be effective. In addition, infants are given single HIV medication for six weeks after birth to decrease the chance of infection further.

CAN I DELIVER MY BABY VAGINALLY IF I HAVE HIV?

During your antenatal care the virus level in your blood will be monitored by a simple blood test. If your levels are high you may benefit from having a caesarean section. If levels are low, vaginal delivery can be continued as normal unless there is another reason for a caesarean section.

CAN I BREASTFEED?

HIV can be transferred in breast milk; therefore, you cannot breastfeed if you are HIV positive.

The prevalence of HIV is high in the Caribbean (1 percent) and the Bahamas (3.1 percent), therefore HIV testing is not only done at the first antenatal visit but also in the third trimester in the event the infection is acquired during pregnancy. Although HIV has no cure, it can be treated in order to delay the conversion to AIDS and also to allow for a prolonged lifespan and good quality of life as well.

Your care will be managed by your obstetric provider and another specialist familiar with HIV. They will work together in deciding on the best care for you and your baby.

SYPHILIS

Syphilis is caused by spiral-like bacteria that can be transmitted to the fetus during pregnancy. If you test positive for syphilis, treatment is with penicillin. If infection is untreated, it can cause a miscarriage, a small baby (*intrauterine growth restriction*), preterm labour, and even fetal death. If infection is acquired in the first trimester during the development of organs, it can result in congenital syphilis. With congenital syphilis the baby can be born with a skin rash, deformed bones and teeth, brain or nerve problems, deafness, or blindness.

Untreated syphilis in the long-term can lead to heart, brain, sight, and nerve damage, with paralysis and even death in the woman.

CHLAMYDIA AND GONORRHOEA

These are both vaginal infections that are caused by bacteria. Women may be unaware that they have these infections, as there are sometimes no symptoms present or it may be missed in screenings. Symptoms include a yellow or pus-like vaginal discharge that is odorless. You may also experience vaginal spotting of blood. Tests for these infections are done routinely in pregnancy through a specialized urine test or by collecting some of the vaginal discharge from the cervix using a cotton-tipped swabbed. If you are positive for chlamydia or gonorrhoea, you will need to be treated with antibiotics. Both of these infections are treatable.

Chlamydia and gonorrhoea if left untreated can have negative effects on your pregnancy. They may cause preterm labour or early rupture of the amniotic sac before term, which can lead to delivery of a premature infant. Transfer of chlamydia and gonorrhoea infection during delivery can cause the infant to have infections of the eyes (*conjunctivitis*), lungs (*pneumonia*), brain (*meningitis*) or bloodstream (*sepsis*). Furthermore, premature infants are susceptible to infections, difficulty breathing and feeding, bleeding in the brain and eyes, and problems with the bowels (just to name a few).

Chlamydia and gonorrhoea if left untreated it can cause problems even after pregnancy as the bacteria can move into the uterus, tubes, and pelvis of the mother, causing a condition known as *pelvic inflammatory disease*. This condition can result in pain and pus in the pelvis with fever, infertility, and chronic pain in the pelvis region that can last months to years.

TRICHOMONIASIS

This infection is caused by a parasite that affects the vagina. It results in increased discharged from the vagina that is green in colour and has a bad odour. Like chlamydia and gonorrhoea, trichomoniasis can also contribute to preterm labour and delivery, early rupture of the water bag, and pelvic inflammatory disease, but to a lesser extent.

Trichomoniasis causes the cervix to become inflamed (and give an appearance similar to the skin of a strawberry). This inflamed cervix can bleed and therefore cause bleeding in pregnancy. The treatment for this infection is with an antibiotic that can be taken by mouth or given as a suppository to insert into the vagina.

HERPES

Herpes is an infection caused by a virus called *herpes simplex virus* (or HSV); there are two types of this virus, HSV-1 and HSV-2. This infection can be transmitted without sexual contact as in the case with oral herpes (cold sores). Genital herpes occurs through sexual contact. Direct contact of the virus to skin or mucous membranes in the genital region or the mouth can result in infection.

In an outbreak of herpes, a crop of small sores is usually seen in the genital region. Fluid in the sores carries the virus. However, even people without a visible sore can still transmit the virus. An outbreak of genital herpes is usually preceded by symptoms that some women can identify, which includes pain or burning in the vaginal area.

If you have genital herpes, it can be transmitted to your baby when passing through the birth canal during labour and delivery or very rarely before labour occurs. It can have many effects if transmitted to your baby, and these include infection of the eyes or brain, a small head (*microcephaly*), and outbreaks of the sores on the skin, mouth, and eyes that can spread to other organs. In some instances, death of your baby can occur. When a newborn baby survives herpes infection, they can still develop learning disabilities, seizures, blindness, and slow achievement of muscle function.

If your very first outbreak of herpes occurs during pregnancy, the chances of transmission to the infant is much higher than if only a second or recurrent outbreak occurs in pregnancy. It is very important for you to tell your healthcare provider if you have genital herpes. An outbreak of herpes is treated using antiviral medications (e.g., *acyclovir* and *valacyclovir*) that will not cure the disease but will reduce the length and severity of the outbreak.

If you are found to have a first or recurrent outbreak at the time of delivery, a caesarean section will be done to decrease the chances of the baby being infected with the herpes virus.

CHAPTER 23

RHESUS INCOMPATIBILITY

RHESUS INCOMPATIBILITY IS a condition that occurs in pregnancy that involves the rhesus antigen. We spoke about this topic a little in the first part of the book, but let's take a closer look. The rhesus antigen (called the *D antigen*) is a small protein that is attached to the surface of red blood cells; if you carry this antigen, you are referred to as being *rhesus positive*. If this antigen is missing, you are *rhesus negative*. The D antigen is spoken about when referring to your blood type (O, A, B, or AB). If a mother has the O blood type and she also has the rhesus D antigen her blood group, she is called O positive. Conversely, if a mother has the O type and does not have the rhesus D antigen, she is O negative.

Rhesus incompatibility only really matters if the mother is rhesus negative but is carrying a fetus that is rhesus positive (i.e., the fetus inherits the D antigen from the father). If the antigen gets into the mother's blood stream (from the fetus's blood), her body sees it as a foreigner and releases proteins made by her immune system known as *anti-D antibodies*. Once these antibodies are produced, the mother is said to be "sensitized." These antibodies do not affect the baby in the pregnancy in which it is produced, but it can affect future pregnancies because it stays in the body forever. For example, if a mother is "sensitized" in her first pregnancy, that baby will be unaffected by the complications of rhesus incompatibility, but in her second pregnancy that baby may be affected. In the affected pregnancies, the antibodies produced can then travel within the blood vessels in the placenta back into the fetus and destroy the baby's red blood cells, which can cause anemia (known as *erythoblastosis fetalis*), and if severe enough can lead to a condition called *hydrops fetalis*, heart failure, or even death in the fetus. In hydrops fetalis the fetus retains water in all the tissues, which makes it difficult to obtain sufficient oxygen to the tissues.

HOW DOES FETAL BLOOD GET INTO THE MOTHER'S BLOOD STREAM? This can happen in a few ways:

1. If there is bleeding at any time during the pregnancy
2. If there is trauma to the abdomen (for example, if mom was hit in the abdomen or fell onto the abdomen)
3. If procedures such as chorionic villi sampling, amniocentesis, or external cephalic version were done
4. During labour and delivery (which is the most common time it happens)
5. If the placenta had to be removed manually after delivery
6. After a miscarriage that was more than 12 weeks gestation or after an ectopic pregnancy

Fetal blood can sometimes get into the mom's circulation because of small, unnoticed bleeds from the placenta that do not cause bleeding from the vagina. So if a procedure needs to be done in pregnancy, it should not be delayed because of fear of rhesus incompatibility, as there are ways to monitor and treat the condition if it occurs. If the mother received a blood transfusion with a rhesus-positive blood group at any time in her life, she would have produced the antibodies that could affect a pregnancy when it occurs.

Rhesus incompatibility is not common; it only happens in less than 2 percent of pregnancies. This is because there are medications that prevent the antibodies from being produced in a rhesus negative mother. Also, if a mother is rhesus negative, a special test called an IDCT is done early in the pregnancy (and sometimes repeated at 28 weeks) in order to know if the anti-D antibodies are in her blood already and how much of it is there. If no antibodies are present, a medication called *anti-D immunoglobulin* is given by injection. This medication destroys any fetal blood cells (with the D antigen) in the mom's blood before the mom's immune system has time to make any antibodies. If antibodies are already there, the medication will not work because it can only prevent them from being formed, not remove them.

WHAT IF MY BODY HAS ALREADY PRODUCED THE ANTIBODIES BEFORE I HAD TIME TO GET THE ANTI-D IMMUNOGLOBULIN?

The levels of the antibodies can be monitored with blood tests during the pregnancy. The baby may also be monitored using ultrasound. If the fetus is anemic then sometimes your doctor may perform a blood transfusion to the fetus to keep the hemoglobin levels up, or the doctor may choose to deliver the baby (even if you are not term in order to avoid complications to the baby).

WHAT WILL HAPPEN AFTER MY BABY IS BORN IF I AM RHESUS NEGATIVE?

A small sample of blood will be taken from the baby to determine the blood group and rhesus status. If the baby is rhesus positive, and you did not have rhesus incompatibility disease during your pregnancy, another dosing of anti-D immunoglobulin is given to you within seventy-two hours of the delivery. Another special test is done on your blood to see if you need additional anti-D (more than the usual dose). If the baby is found to be rhesus negative then no anti-D immunoglobulin is needed after delivery.

Antibody levels will be measured in every pregnancy that you have if you are rhesus negative. Even if you have received the anti-D immunoglobulin in a prior pregnancy, if you are not sensitized you will receive it in another pregnancy because the effects of the anti-D immunoglobulin only last for about twelve weeks.

DOWN'S SYNDROME AND OTHER FETAL ANEUPLOIDIES

AN *ANEUPLOIDY* IS a condition where there are an abnormal number of chromosomes present in the fetus. Genes are carried in structures called *chromosomes*. Each cell has an area that carries this genetic material called the *nucleus*. The nucleus has twenty-three pairs of chromosome (half of each pair is inherited from each parent).

TRISOMY 21 (DOWN'S SYNDROME)

One of the most common aneuploidies is Down's syndrome (also known as trisomy 21), where there is an extra copy of chromosome number 21. Babies with Down's syndrome can live outside the womb, but they will have varying levels of cognitive delay (very mild to severe) and some may have other abnormalities such as heart problems. This condition causes specific physical features; the facial features are most prominent with small, upward slanting eyes with extra folds of skin, low muscle tone, and a single crease going across the palm of the hand. The risk of Down's syndrome (DS) increases with the age of the mother, especially over thirty-five years old. For example, at age twenty-five the risk is about a one in twelve thousand chance of having a baby with Down's compared with a one in eighty-five risk at age forty years old. However, 80 percent of the cases of Down's occur in mothers younger than thirty-five years old. Down's syndrome may be diagnosed during pregnancy using a quad screen with amniocentesis or chorionic villi sampling (which we spoke about in chapter 2) or after delivery by the external features, along with chromosome testing (called *karyotyping)*. There is also a combination of blood tests and ultrasound tests done in the first and second trimester that together can identify 95 percent of the cases of Down's syndrome.

IF I HAD A BABY WITH DOWN'S SYNDROME BEFORE, CAN IT OCCUR IN ANOTHER PREGNANCY?

Yes, but this is rare. There is one type of Down's syndrome that can be hereditary (in about 1 percent of cases). Outside of the rare hereditary type, the chance of having another baby with Down's is about one in one hundred up until the age of forty years.

TRISOMY 18 (EDWARD'S SYNDROME)

This type of aneuploidy is far less common than Down's syndrome. It is caused by an extra chromosome 18. Most infants with trisomy 18 die before birth in the second or third trimester. The babies that survive to delivery may die within a few months to years of birth. Girls are more likely to survive than boys. The children that survive have significant delays in their development. Trisomy 18 can be diagnosed similarly to Down's syndrome with a combination of testing in the second and first trimester, amniocentesis (or chorionic villi sampling), and ultrasound.

They have specific features and serious health problems, including: Babies tend to have a clenched fist, deformed feet (that are curved like the bottom of a rocking chair), problems with feeding, cleft palate, a hole in the heart, a small head and jaw, a weak cry, and defects in other organs. Children with this condition require lifelong care well into adulthood. They can live to their twenties or thirties.

TRISOMY 13 (PATAU SYNDROME)

These infants have an extra copy of chromosome 13 and have severe health problems involving almost every organ and abnormal physical features. Many of them fail to grow and gain weight and have severe feeding difficulties.

Ears and facial features are abnormal, and areas of skin on the scalp may be missing. Extra fingers and toes are not uncommon, along with undescended testes in boys and strangely shaped uteri in girls. Also, there may be incomplete brain development leading to profound mental retardation and delays in development. Half of the babies die within thirty days of life and others survive to be between age one and age ten.

If your child is diagnosed with any of these conditions before or after birth, your healthcare provider may suggest genetic counselling, and there are also support groups that you can join. Caring for a special needs child is challenging, and it is important that you have all the emotional and physical support that you can get. Every child is precious and is a gift from God.

"Children are a gift from the LORD; they are a reward
from him."

—Psalm 127:3 (NLT)

CHAPTER 25

ORGAN TRANSPLANT

CONCEPTION IS NOT advised within the first year after organ transplant surgery. Although a vaginal delivery is not contraindicated, a discussion with your healthcare team will review the optimum mode of delivery to suit your case. If possible, it would be beneficial to deliver in a unit where a transplant surgeon can be present in a scheduled or unscheduled delivery.

RENAL TRANSPLANT

In the case of a renal transplant, your doctor would check your kidney function and for any diseases that may be present. *Teratogenic* (harmful to the developing fetus) medications would have to be discontinued prior to pregnancy. You may require medications to help prevent a deep vein thrombosis depending on your renal function. You may also require an erythropoietin-stimulating agent (which helps to increase your red blood cell count). Your care should be coordinated by an experienced obstetrician and a multidisciplinary team of doctors. If you have donated a kidney, your doctor may recommend aspirin during your pregnancy.

PANCREAS TRANSPLANT

If the pancreas is transplanted alone or you have undergone a pancreas and kidney transplant, both organs will have to be monitored throughout your pregnancy. Your provider may decide to deliver you by caesarean delivery, but vaginal delivery is not contraindicated.

LIVER TRANSPLANT
It is not known if pregnancy affects the liver transplant. However, a liver transplant is not a contraindication to a vaginal delivery.

HEART AND LUNG TRANSPLANTS
Cardiac and pulmonary transplant patients have to be assessed individually. With a lung transplant, your pregnancy risk may be increased when compared to other transplant patients. Your pregnancy may be more challenging to manage. However, this is not a contraindication to a vaginal delivery.

MEDICATIONS IN TRANSPLANT RECIPIENTS
People who have received organ transplants are required to take medications called *immunosuppressive drugs* that decrease the response of their immune systems so that their bodies do not reject the transplanted organ. Not all of these medications are safe in pregnancy. Table 5 notes some of the more common medications that are used in persons with transplants and their effects on the fetus. However, a discussion should be made with both your transplant physicians and your obstetrician before and during your pregnancy for them to come up with the best plan for you.

Table 5

Medication	**Effects on your baby during pregnancy**
Prednisone	May slow down growth and result in a baby born with a low birth weight.
Tacrolimus	May cause diabetes.
Azathioprine	May cause your baby's growth to be slow or cause abnormalities in organs.
Cyclosporine	May slow down your baby's growth and cause early labour and delivery.

DIALYSIS DURING PREGNANCY

Women who are on dialysis have a reduced rate of pregnancy. The effects of dialysis on pregnancy include miscarriage, preterm labour, premature rupture of membranes, placental abruption, and intrauterine death.

If you are on hemodialysis, you may have to increase the frequency of your hemodialysis. You may have to continue to monitor your fluid intake.

If you have had a renal transplant, you may be advised to wait one to two years after transplantation to minimize the risk to the fetus from the immunosuppression drugs and to allow time for the manifestation and resolution from any adverse reactions such as graft-versus-host disease (a condition in which the body attacks and rejected the transplanted organ).

The pregnancy will not have any negative impact on your transplant if your renal function is near normal. If your function is abnormal or you have hypertension you have an increased chance of developing complications such as preeclampsia, rejection of the transplant, and infections. Problems with the baby's growth in the womb and possible early delivery can also occur.

Your healthcare provider may manage your pregnancy with other specialists. They may monitor you for infections in the urine, proteins, and some types of infections, such as *cytomegalovirus*. Your fetus may be monitored with ultrasound. Your provider will monitor your immunosuppression regimen. Antibiotics may be given as prophylaxis for any surgical procedure. Moreover, steroids may be required in labour if you have been on steroids.

C H A P T E R 2 6

PULMONARY DISEASES

PNEUMONIA

COMMUNITY-ACQUIRED PNEUMONIA IS the most common form of pneumonia in pregnancy. Bacterial organisms such as *Streptococcus pneumoniae, Haemophilus influenzae,* and *Mycoplasma pneumoniae* are the most common bacterial organisms responsible for pneumonia during pregnancy. Viral respiratory infections, including varicella, influenza, and severe acute respiratory syndrome, can be associated with pneumonia in pregnancy.

Pneumonia in pregnancy is linked to increased morbidity (illness) and mortality compared with nonpregnant women. If you have diseases such as asthma and anemia, it increases your risk of contracting pneumonia in pregnancy. Effects of pneumonia in pregnancy include respiratory failure in the mother and fetal complications such as low birth weight and increased risk for early birth.

Beta-lactam and macrolide antibiotics (e.g., penicillins, cephalosporins, and erythromycins) are considered safe in pregnancy and are effective for most community-acquired pneumonia in pregnancy. Antiviral and respiratory therapies can reduce maternal morbidity and mortality from viral pneumonia.

Influenza vaccination can reduce the prevalence of respiratory hospitalisations among pregnant women during influenza season. *Pneumocystis* pneumonia can be detrimental if you are immunocompromised (meaning you have an immune system with cells that cannot fight off infection very well). Prevention and treatment of *Pneumocystis* pneumonia with *trimethoprim/sulfamethoxazole* is effective in reducing this risk.

Early diagnosis and supportive care is important to reduce the complications of pneumonia. Prevention with vaccination if you are at an increased risk may also reduce the occurrence or severity of the disease.

PCP (*PNEUMOCYSTIS CARINII* PNEUMONIA)

This is the most common opportunistic infection in AIDs (opportunistic infections are those that invade the body when the immune system is weak). It is treated with Bactrim®. Mothers with HIV that have a low CD4 count may be given prophylaxis for PCP.

TUBERCULOSIS

Tuberculosis onset can sometimes be slow with symptoms that include cough, blood in the secretions coughed, weight loss, or perfuse sweating at night. It affects the lungs but can also affect other parts of the body, such as the lymph nodes, eyes, nervous system, bones, liver, and spleen.

A Mantoux test (which observes your skin reaction to a solution placed just under the skin on the inner arm) and a chest X-ray will be done if it is suspected that you have tuberculosis.

Congenital tuberculosis is rare, and there is little evidence that it has a negative effect on pregnancy, but tuberculosis should be treated if diagnosed in pregnancy. The disease may be treated with one or more drugs. Within two weeks of commencing treatment, you will usually become noninfectious; however, treatment is continued for several months.

CYSTIC FIBROSIS

Cystic fibrosis is a genetic disorder that affects mucus production and the movement of water and salts across the skin's surface. As a result you may have difficulty with recurrent lung infections and failure of the lungs. Problems with the pancreas may lead to diabetes. Maternal morbidity and mortality may be affected by the amount of lung dysfunction.

Some of the complications for a pregnant woman with cystic fibrosis include congestive heart failure, decline in respiratory states, increased risk of gestational diabetes, and poor weight gain. Other issues may include a preterm delivery and poor growth of the fetus. Your management in pregnancy should include consultation with a nutritionist and a high-risk maternal fetal specialist.

If you have severe lung disease, which may be a result of conditions such as *kyphoscoliosis* and *scleroderma*, it may be important to oversee your care with a pulmonologist.

SARCOIDOSIS

This is a disorder that does not affect many pregnant women. It is a disease that affects many systems, such as the skin, eyes, joints, and nervous system. It is diagnosed by chest X-ray with the findings of lymph nodes. A blood test checking for levels of angiotensin-converting enzymes may also help with the diagnosis. The disorder may regress during pregnancy. You should avoid vitamin D supplementation, which may worsen increased levels of calcium noted in this disorder. If your provider decides that steroids are needed in the treatment of this illness, you may require steroids at the time of delivery and in the postpartum period.

ASTHMA

Asthma is a condition in which the airway passages in the lungs (the *bronchial tree*) constricts (narrows) affecting adequate transfer of oxygen from the lungs into the blood. It also results in retention of gases that should be exhaled (e.g., carbon dioxide). Asthma is usually diagnosed in children; however, it can first occur during adulthood and is more common in people with *atopy*, which includes eczema and allergic rhinitis (nasal allergies). Asthma causes shortness of breath with wheezing. Triggers for asthmatic attacks are many, but they include pet dander, dust, pollen, smoke, and aspirin. When an attack is severe, if not treated it can lead to failure of the lungs and even death. Asthmatic attacks can increase in pregnancy or remain the same. If you have asthma, it is important to take your long-term medications and short-term relievers, such as salbutamol (Ventolin®). Discuss your symptoms and medications with your healthcare provider, as medications such as oral steroids should not be taken in the first trimester because of its association with cleft palate.

CHAPTER 27

INSOMNIA

Insomnia (trouble sleeping) is a common occurrence as pregnancy progresses. It may be frustrating, especially if you have to work and take care of your household during the day. Please find some tips for dealing with insomnia in pregnancy.

- Eat your food slowly and don't eat close to bedtime to avoid acid reflux and a full stomach while you sleep.
- Avoid caffeine and chocolate especially close to bedtime as they can keep you up.
- Do not drink before bedtime. Drink your fluids during the early evening to cut down on bathroom runs after you've fallen asleep.
- Get some daily pregnancy exercise, but not too close to bedtime.
- Make sure your head is clear. If you have worries that are keeping you up nights, talk about them with a friend, your partner, and God (in prayer). Get everything off your mind before you lie down. Journaling (writing your worries down) is often helpful.
- Establish a bedtime routine. Try to go to sleep and get up at the same time every day.
- Relax. Consider using a warm bath, a cup of warm milk, or a relaxing prenatal massage to put yourself in a sleepy state.
- Make sure your environment is comfortable. If you're uncomfortable, you won't sleep. Check the temperature of your room, the condition of your mattress and pillows, and make sure room is clean and organized and smells good.

- Only use your bed for sex and sleep. Do daytime activities outside the bed, such as eating, reading, or bill paying.
- Don't use sleep aids (unless specifically directed by your doctor). If you're not sleeping, get up. If you're not asleep after twenty to thirty minutes of trying, do a small, short task and then try to go to sleep again.

Instead of aiming for a particular number of sleep hours, look at how you are feeling on the hours that you are sleeping.

HERE ARE SOME SCRIPTURE TO MEDITATE ON WHEN YOU'RE HAVING TROUBLE SLEEPING:

"It is in vain that you rise up early and go late to rest, eating the bread of anxious toil; for he gives to his beloved sleep."

—PSALM 127:2 (ESV)

"When you lie down, you will not be afraid; when you lie down, your sleep will be sweet."

—PROVERBS 3:24 (NIV)

"You will lie down, with no one to make you afraid, and many will court your favor."

—JOB 11:19 (NIV)

"I will both lie down in peace, and sleep: for You alone, O LORD, make me dwell in safety."

—PSALM 4:8 (NKJV)

*"At this I awoke and looked around. My sleep had been
pleasant to me."*

—Jeremiah 31:26 (NIV)

DIZZINESS

DIZZINESS IS A common complaint in pregnancy that has several possible causes. One cause may be that the progesterone causes a relaxation of the blood vessels that may cause a reduction in blood pressure. Another cause is low blood sugar levels that may occur as your body adapts to changes in your metabolism (and the glucose it transfers to the fetus for energy).

Women who have low haemoglobin levels and varicose veins may be more likely to experience dizziness than others. During the second half of pregnancy, dizziness may be caused by your growing uterus putting pressure on blood vessels, such as the *vena cava* (a large vein that carries blood from your lower body to your heart).

How can I prevent dizziness when I am pregnant?

- Avoid standing for long periods. While standing, make sure that you keep your feet moving to help increase circulation.
- Avoid lying down or sitting for prolonged periods of time.
- Get up slowly from either sitting or lying down.
- Eat regularly. Do not skip meals and try to snack throughout the day. Keep hydrated.
- Avoid lying on your back once you reach the middle of your second trimester.
- Wear loose, comfortable clothing to avoid affecting circulation.
- Avoid hot baths or showers.
- Avoid constricting or tight clothes.

There are also a few things you can do to help relieve the feeling that you are going to faint:

- Let someone near you know that you are not feeling well.
- Stop whatever activity you are engaged in, especially if you are driving, cooking, bathing, or operating machinery.
- Sit or lie down and lower your head.
- Take deep breaths.
- Loosen any tight clothing.
- Open windows and move towards circulating air.

You should also contact your healthcare provider immediately if you have persistent dizziness or dizziness accompanied by blurred vision, headaches, chest pain, or heart palpitations.

C H A P T E R   2 9

OTHER CONDITIONS

THERE ARE MANY other chronic conditions that women can have that must be managed during pregnancy, often by a team of healthcare providers. In this chapter, we want to give mention to a few more.

LUPUS

This is a systemic connective tissue disorder that is more common in Afro-Caribbean women. It is charaterised by remission and flares. The cause is not known, but there are many theories. It is classified as an autoimmune disorder, which include conditions in which the body produces antibodies that in turn attack varying organs in the body. Lupus can affect almost every organ system in the body. Pregnancy increases the likelihood of a flare significantly and can also be difficult to diagnose as many of the features occur in normal pregnancy. If you have lupus, it is important to see your healthcare provider before you get pregnant to discuss your risks, optimal timing for conception, pregnancy management and possible fetal outcomes.

THYROID DISEASE

Thyroid disorders are common in women in the reproductive age group. Women can have an overactive thyroid gland that produces too much thyroid hormones (known as hyperthyroidism) or an underactive gland (known as hypothyroidism). Thyroid hormones are responsible for maintaining a balance in the functioning of other organs in the body. The most common cause of hyperthyroidism is Grave's disease and for hypothyroidism is Hashimoto's thyroiditis, which are both autoimmune disorders. When the gland is not functioning well, it can lead to pregnancy complications such as; pre-eclampsia/eclampsia, hyperemesis gravidarum, preterm delivery and pregnancy loss. The fetus may develop growth restriction, dysfunction of their thyroid gland or heart failure. If you have thyroid disease it is important to have a discussion with your healthcare provider so that appropriate treatment and monitoring can be done to decrease the chances of complications in your pregnancy.

ANTIPHOSPHOLIPID ANTIBODY SYNDROME

This is an autoimmune condition in which the body produces various types of antibodies that can cause harm. Antibodies generally are helpful in fighting off disease and strengthening the immune system. However, during pregnancy the antibodies in this condition can lead to blood clots, recurrent miscarriages and pre-eclampsia/eclampsia. Medications are available that can decrease the chances of these complications occurring during pregnancy.

GALLBLADDER DISEASE

The gallbladder is a small organ responsible for heping to digest consumed fats. Gallbladder disease is not very common in pregnancy, however, gallstones are common and can be found in women before pregnancy or they can form during. Some will resolve postpartum. The symptoms are similar to non-pregnant women, with nausea, vomiting and indigestion. Complications of gallstones include inflammation of the gallbladder or pancreas. If the inflammation becomes severe and symptoms do not resolve, surgery may be required during pregnancy.

SECTION 4
SOCIAL ISSUES AND COPING WITH LOSS

C H A P T E R   3 0

COPING WITH LOSS

MISCARRIAGE, ECTOPIC PREGNANCY, AND STILLBIRTH

MISCARRIAGE: A LOSS that occurs before 20 weeks in some countries and 24–28 weeks in other countries. Generally, below the age of viability (which we spoke about in the first chapter) is considered a miscarriage. A miscarriage may be as stressful as a loss at term.

Ectopic Pregnancy: A type of miscarriage in which the embryo (or fetus) is located outside of the cavity of the uterus. It usually occurs in the first or early second trimester. If it occurs after the age of viability, it is then referred to as an abdominal pregnancy. It is treated either with medications or by removing the pregnancy by surgery. Ectopic pregnancies most commonly occur in the fallopian tubes, which can tear when stretched and cause bleeding within the abdomen that can lead to death of the mother if severe and not treated. Ectopic pregnancies cannot be salvaged (even when a heartbeat is detected) because a pregnancy needs to be within the uterus to develop normally. Very rarely an abdominal pregnancy may make it to viability, but these cases are still associated with a high risk of death of the mother and fetus or infection, even when caught early and the baby is delivered by C-section.

Stillborn or Neonatal Death: A stillborn is as an infant who had died in the womb after the age of viability (usually 22 or 24 weeks). A neonatal death is an infant who dies less than twenty-eight days after birth. These deaths are usually unexpected.

The most common cause of the above losses may be problems with the baby's growth (*intrauterine growth restriction*), placental abruption, mothers

185

with uncontrolled diabetes, or prematurity or complications of prematurity, such as infections, problems with the intestines (*necrotizing enterocolitis*), bleeding in the brain (*intraventricular haemorrhage*), or lung problems such as respiratory distress syndrome or infections.

LOSS OF A MULTIPLE

The loss of one or more babies in multiple gestation is complicated. You may have a lengthened grieving process compared to someone who has lost a single baby.

THE GRIEVING PROCESS

It is important to note that grief is a very personal and case-specific process. No book or expert can tell you how to grieve or what your process will be like. All losses, however, have the phases of grieving in common that many parents experience.

1. *Shock and numbness*: You may feel stunned, your emotions may seem unstable, or you may have difficulty concentrating or making decisions. At times you may feel overwhelmed, anxious, or unconfident.
2. *Searching and yearning:* You may have physical symptoms that include fatigue, headaches, and change in appetite. You may dream about your baby. If you have children that have survived, it may be a challenge to care for them, as you may remember the missing child to be cared for. If there are no survivors, the body changes, including milk let-down, may serve as a painful reminder of your loss.
3. *Anger*: You may be angry with yourself, angry with your physician, and angry with God for your loss. You may not understand or be able to express your feelings.
4. *Depression*: You may feel that your day-to-day activities are without any pleasure. This emotion may be a normal part of the process, but if it lasts longer than six months or you ever feel like hurting someone

(including yourself), this is a medical emergency and you should seek help immediately.

5. *Acceptance:* You may acknowledge and come to terms with the loss of your child.

WHAT ARE THE OPTIONS IF MY BABY DIES IN UTERO OR CHILDBIRTH?

Know that the choices are dependent on you. You may opt to hold your infant or wash and dress your infant. You may choose not to hold your baby.

A postmortem exam may be valuable to help find out the cause of your baby's death. This may be helpful if the cause is due to a congenital defect or genetic issues. This information may be helpful in a future pregnancy. Sometimes a postmortem is unable to determine the cause of your baby's death.

Use sources of support that are available locally or internationally. Losing your child is a very painful experience.

TRYING TO CONCEIVE AGAIN

Most people who have suffered a loss of some type often make the decision to try to conceive again. This may be a difficult decision, and the subsequent pregnancy is often emotionally challenging. But in time, you develop the ability to cope with another pregnancy and cope with the loss of the previous child.

The time to start trying is usually up to you and your partner (after a discussion with your healthcare provider). Ensure that any chronic conditions that may have impacted your pregnancy are stable and optimized. Consider evaluating your emotional and financial status to make sure they are stable to avoid incurring additional stress.

It is important to understand that the subsequent child will not replace the child that you lost. You should also recognize that it is okay to have another child and it is okay for you to be happy. A perinatal loss (during or within weeks after delivery) has the potential to have a dramatic impact on both parents, their relationship with each other, and possibly their relationship with other children.

AS YOU COPE WITH YOUR LOSS MEDITATE ON THE SCRIPTURE BELOW:

"The LORD will give you prosperity in the land he swore to your ancestors to give you, blessing you with many children."

—DEUTERONOMY 28:11 (NLT)

"They that sow in tears shall reap in joy."

—PSALM 126:5 (KJV)

"Cast thy burden upon the LORD, and he shall sustain thee: he shall never suffer the righteous to be moved."

—PSALM 55:22 (KJV)

"Come unto me, all ye that labor and are heavy laden, and I will give you rest."

—MATTHEW 11:28 (KJV)

"Casting all your care upon him; for he careth for you."

—1 PETER 5:7 (KJV)

"Wait on the LORD: be of good courage, and he shall strengthen thine heart: wait, I say, on the LORD."

—PSALM 27:14 (KJV)

"Blessed are they that mourn: for they shall be comforted."

—MATTHEW 5:4 (KJV)

"This is my comfort in my affliction: for thy word hath quickened me."

—PSALM 119:50 (KJV)

CHAPTER 31

SOCIAL ISSUES

DOMESTIC VIOLENCE

DOMESTIC VIOLENCE IS defined (by the Home Office department of the Government of the United Kingdom) as "any incident or pattern of controlling, coercive or threatening behaviour, violence, or abuse (psychological, physical, sexual, financial, or emotional) between adults who are or have been intimate partners or family members, regardless of gender or sexuality. This definition includes those aged 16 or over." Domestic violence in pregnancy is considered intimate-partner violence. Abuse can take different forms:

PHYSICAL ABUSE

Physical effects are often in areas of the body that are covered and hidden (i.e., breasts, arms, and abdomen). Shaking, smacking, punching, kicking, starving, tying up, stabbing, suffocation, throwing things at you as weapons, female genital mutilation (where the female genitals are deliberately cut or injured, without a medical reason), and "honor violence" (which is domestic violence that is often condoned by families or communities or certain groups) are examples of physical abuse.

SEXUAL ABUSE

Forced sex, forced prostitution, ignoring religious prohibitions about sex, refusal to practice safe sex, sexual insults, and or preventing breastfeeding are all forms of sexual abuse.

Psychological Abuse

Intimidating, insulting, isolating you from friends and family, criticizing you, treating you as an inferior, and threatening to hurt your children or take them away are examples of psychological abuse.

Financial Abuse

Stopping you from working, discouraging your efforts to find work or study, refusing to give you money, requesting an explanation of how every penny is spent, making you beg for money, gambling, and/or not paying bills are examples of financial abuse.

Emotional Abuse

Swearing, undermining your confidence, making you feel unattractive/ unworthy, calling you names, or corroding your independence are examples of emotional abuse.

Remember, you must not listen to the lies of the enemy about your character spoken to you through people. You are precious to God.

> *"Since you are precious and honored in my sight, and because*
> *I love you, I will give people in exchange for you, nations in*
> *exchange for your life."*
>
> — Isaiah 43:4 (NIV)

Many women experience domestic abuse or domestic violence at some point in their lives. It is estimated that one-quarter of women encounter domestic violence. Abuse may be physical, sexual, emotional, or psychological. Approximately one out of three cases starts or worsens in pregnancy, and existing abuse may get worse during pregnancy or after giving birth.

Domestic abuse during pregnancy puts you and your fetus in a dangerous situation. It increases the risk of miscarriage, infection, premature birth, injury or death to the baby, and death to you. It is important for you to recognize the signs of abuse and watch for any of the examples listed above.

GETTING HELP

If you are pregnant and being abused, help is available. You should not hesitate to talk to:

- Your healthcare provider
- Social workers
- Police
- Domestic violence help lines
- God

MEDITATE ON THESE SCRIPTURES:

"Husbands, love your wives and do not be harsh with them."

—COLOSSIANS 3:19 (NIV)

"The LORD examines the righteous, but the wicked, those who love violence, he hates with a passion."

—PSALM 11:5 (NIV)

"Let no corrupt communication proceed out of your mouth, but that which is good to the use of edifying, that it may minister grace unto the hearers."

—EPHESIANS 4:29 (KJV)

"He shall redeem their soul from deceit and violence: and precious shall their blood be in his sight."

—Psalm 72:14 (KJV)

"The LORD also will be a refuge for the oppressed, a refuge in times of trouble."

—Psalm 9:9 (KJV)

ALCOHOL AND DRUGS IN PREGNANCY

Your baby is connected to you through the umbilical cord. As a result, whatever you put in your system also gets into your baby's system. Some drugs have toxic effects on the baby, causing problems such as malformations, fetal loss, problems with growth, early labour, dependency on the drugs, neurodevelopmental issues, and possible complications with you, the mother.

Alcohol

We know that alcohol can have an effect on your baby, but we do not know exactly how many drinks it takes for this effect to happen. With this in mind, we recommend that you refrain from drinking during pregnancy. Alcohol may increase the risk of heart defects in the infant.

Fetal alcohol syndrome is due to alcohol consumption in pregnancy and consists of abnormalities with the baby's face, growth restriction, mental retardation, problems with the reproductive tract and the appendages (limbs), and problems with the way the baby's heart forms.

MARIJUANA

The use of marijuana (also known as *cannabis* or *weed*) in pregnancy can increase substances such as carbon dioxide and carbon monoxide in the blood, which in turn may affect the oxygen supply to the fetus. This may affect growth of the fetus and later neurological development. Some studies have shown that children exposed to marijuana in the womb are more likely to show issues with problem-solving skills, memory, and attention. If you use marijuana, your risk of miscarriage is also increased.

TOBACCO SMOKING

Smoking in pregnancy is fairly common. However, smoking is detrimental for the mother and the fetus. Even second- and thirdhand smoke have been shown to have negative effects on the baby in the short term and long term. Numerous toxins are found in cigarette smoke, including nicotine, arsenic, tar, lead, and carbon monoxide. These toxins decrease the amount of oxygen that can get to your baby. Complications that can occur include preterm labour, growth restriction, a low birth weight in your baby, placental abruption, and placental previa. Your baby may even have to stay in the hospital longer than usual if you smoke during your pregnancy. Furthermore, your infant has a greater chance of dying from *sudden infant death syndrome* (SIDS).

When you quit smoking, your baby benefits in many ways. It will get more oxygen, which helps with growth and development. You will decrease the chance of your child having asthma and bronchitis. You will also decrease his or her risk of heart disease later in life. Electronic cigarettes have been designed, but these also are harmful and should not be used. Smoking can make it difficult to become pregnant or may cause an ectopic pregnancy.

LSD AND PCP

These drugs cause hallucinations (making you see things and have sensations and perceptions that are not real) that may cause you to harm yourself. If this happens and you are pregnant, you could also harm the fetus. These drugs can affect fetal development and the baby can experience withdrawal symptoms when born.

ECSTASY

Ecstasy, or MDMA (which stands for *3,4-methylenedioxymethamphetamine*), is a synthetic drug that has been shown to impact the brain and motor developmental of infants.

COCAINE

This drug has the potential to have a profound effect on your pregnancy, including possible birth defects with prolonged use and miscarriage. Later in the pregnancy the drug has possibility to cause a placental abruption, high blood pressure, poor fetal growth, and preterm labour. The infant also has a chance of being born addicted to this drug and may have withdrawal symptoms and other long-term effects.

HEROIN

Heroin use during pregnancy is linked with medical and obstetrical complications and may result in both acute and chronic abnormalities in neonates. Malnutrition, hepatitis, lung complications, sexually transmitted infections, preeclampsia, and bleeding are the most common maternal complications. Complications with the baby include fetal death, intrauterine growth retardation, prematurity, and withdrawal symptoms. Methadone during pregnancy may be used, but it also has some similar long-term effects such as long-lasting drug-induced syndrome, characterized by growth retardation, delayed motor development, and behaviour abnormalities.

CAFFEINE

Caffeine is a stimulant and diuretic. It increases your heart rate and causes you to void more often. Caffeine in pregnancy is a difficult topic, as we do not know exactly how much caffeine consumption it requires to have a negative effect on the fetus. Animal studies, as opposed to human studies, have shown an increase in negative outcomes such as growth issues, early labour, and birth defects. We do know that more than 300 mg daily possibly increases the risk of miscarriage and that it takes the fetus longer to get rid of the caffeine compared to you. With this in mind, we recommend that you minimize your caffeine intake as much as possible. We suspect that one 11-oz cup of coffee a day (200 mg of caffeine) is probably safe in pregnancy.

If you use any of the substances mentioned in this section, make sure to notify your healthcare provider. If you are interested in stopping, your provider would be the best person to give guidance and resources that will be most helpful in your journey. Be encouraged and know that even if it is challenging to stop the use of your substance of choice, your baby will be grateful and so will you.

CAN WE AFFORD THIS PREGNANCY?

If we can't how can we get there? Usually couples save up for big purchases, such as a house or car, and pregnancy and childbirth should be viewed as a big purchase. So below are some tips in preparing financially for a pregnancy. Preparation may decrease your stress associated with this life-changing process.

BUDGET REVIEW

Prepregnancy is definitely a good time to sit down and have a review of your budget (or at least in early pregnancy). Look to see if your income exceeds your expenditures. Review and cut out or cut down any unnecessary expenses. Consider paying off or down any debt such as credit cards, car loans, student loans, etc.

Consider the extra expenses per month associated with a child and redo your budget including this cost. Consider setting aside these extra funds for three months to one year.

EMPLOYMENT

As a team you have to decide (if you both are employed) whether one partner is going to stay home or return to work. If one parent is going to stay home, you have to look at your budget on one income. Before you make this leap, it may be helpful to practice living off one income and setting the other one aside to see if this will work for your household.

ANTENATAL CARE AND DELIVERY COST

INSURANCE

If possible you may want to consider signing up for insurance with maternity benefits at least one year before you conceive. Check different plans and compare to see who has the best benefits and best premiums. Find out what your deductible is per year (the amount that you would have to pay before the insurance pays its portion). Find out what your percentage of contribution is once the deductible has been paid.

Try to save your deductible in advance as much as possible and set aside additional funds to cover that portion that would be your responsibility. If you are paying cash for your services, you may consider checking on the cost of lab fees, hospital fees, and paediatrician and healthcare provider fees.

Lab fees and hospital fees: discounted fees may be available for cash-paying patients.

Provider costs: obstetrician and paediatrician; may be different for vaginal delivery and caesarean section. It is important to ask about the cost of each option and be prepared in the event that a surgical procedure is available. Most providers may have a payment plan so that most, if not all, of the delivery can be paid for before delivery. This allows you to focus on other costs.

Anaesthesiology cost: It is important to consider the cost of an epidural or spinal. Although you may not plan to have a pain intervention, you may change your mind or circumstances may mandate that you use an anaesthesiologist's services.

Miscellaneous: It is also important to make an allowance for items associated with birth, such as clothes, milk, pampers, a car seat, and maternity clothes. With this in mind, it may be good idea to have some funds set aside for emergencies or miscellaneous funds at time of delivery. Although you may not be able to contain your excitement, consider waiting for your baby shower and then only purchasing items that were not purchased that you need. Consider obtaining items that are secondhand, such as baby furniture.

It is important to consider, too, policies for maternity leave and sick leave if you are employed. Some ladies also have complications during pregnancy that prevent them from continuing employment during pregnancy. Therefore, it is important to take this into consideration and how it could possibly affect your household finances.

Taking time to consider these issues will undoubtedly be beneficial and decrease the potential financial stress that could be associated with a pregnancy. It also gives you an opportunity to prepare and plan so that you can enjoy your pregnancy.

APPENDIX A: COMMON QUESTIONS YOU ALWAYS WANTED TO ASK

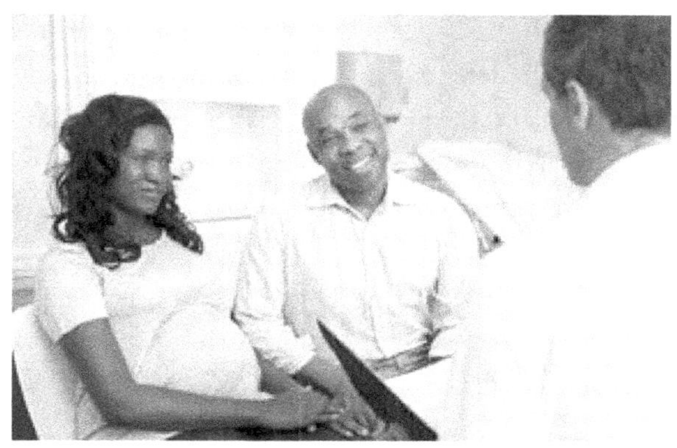

No question is a silly question; every question has merit.

Can I drink wine or other alcoholic beverages? No. Alcohol should not be consumed during pregnancy as it can lead to a condition called fetal alcohol syndrome (FAS). There is no clear correlation on the amount of alcohol consumed, the gestation it is consumed at, and the occurrence of FAS, therefore no amount should be consumed.

Can I go on water slides? No. With advancing pregnancy, the sudden plunge into the water can lead to a transfer of pressure forces to the uterus that could cause interruption in the placenta and bleeding. It can also cause premature labour or trauma to the baby. Also, you can injure yourself due to the increasing imbalance experienced by pregnant women. However, tubing is calm; still water is okay. If you inadvertently go on a water slide, being unaware of an early first trimester pregnancy, it is likely not to cause any harm.

Can I go on a roller coaster? No. Roller coasters, because of the frequent sudden movements and changes in altitude, can possibly cause placental abruption and harm to your baby. Also it can lead to extreme nausea and vomiting during or after a ride.

Can I go in a hot tub? No. Hot tubs can cause an excessive increase in body temperature (*hyperthermia*) that can affect a developing fetus in the first trimester and lead to birth defects, so they should be avoided. A hot bath is better if you need to relax aching muscles, as the temperature begins to cool down, preventing hyperthermia, as opposed to hot tubs in which the water circulates and maintains a temperature of 102 to 104 degrees Fahrenheit.

Can I go in a pool? Yes. Swimming is often relaxing for pregnant women and can be a form of low-impact exercising during pregnancy. However, you should not do any diving while pregnant.

Why am I spitting all the time? This is called *ptyalism* or hypersalivation. It is not uncommon in pregnancy.

Can I dye my hair or perm my hair? Yes. Getting a perm does not affect the course of your pregnancy. Hair dye can be permanent or semipermanent. These do not appear to affect your pregnancy, as it cannot reach the fetus since only a very little is absorbed into the scalp. The minimal fumes you are exposed to at the hair salon from these products do not affect your pregnancy either.

Can I get a pedicure or manicure? Yes. These are quite safe in pregnancy. Acrylic nail use and fingernail polish is also safe.

Can I drink coffee or tea? Yes. But you should minimize your caffeine intake as much as possible. We suspect that one 11-oz cup of coffee a day (200 mg of caffeine) is probably safe in pregnancy. If you can do without it, then do so. Teas can be consumed, but take this with a grain of salt. Herbal teas can be safe if commercially made; however, unregulated herbal teas may be harmful to your pregnancy. Some examples of safe herbal teas are red raspberry leaf, peppermint leaf, and ginger root teas.

Can I drive? Yes. You should always wear you seat belt when in a vehicle (driving or not). It is important as your abdomen gets bigger that you wear your seat belt correctly to prevent injuries. Ensure that the lap belt and shoulder belt are fitting snuggly across your body. The lap belt should be under your abdomen, never across it. Also, do not place the shoulder strap under your arm; it should be across the shoulder. Avoid long driving times without stopping to get of out the car and walk around. Long driving can increase your risk for deep vein thrombosis.

Can I smoke weed (marijuana)? No. Smoking can affect your baby's development and decreased the amount of oxygen getting to your baby. There may also be some link to issues with problem solving and cognitive thinking in children who were exposed to marijuana in the uterus.

What can I take for a cold, headache, or fever? Colds (upper respiratory tract infections) are often due to viruses and are self-limiting and resolve without treatment. However, if symptoms are troublesome, certain medication can be used. Headaches and fevers can accompany the common cold, but they can also be symptoms of other serious illnesses. A healthcare provider should check symptoms that are severe or not resolving. See appendix B for a list of medications you can use for the symptoms of a cold, headache, or fever, including pain relievers and fever reducers. Note that most of these medications should be avoided in the first trimester.

Can I see a chiropractor? Yes. However, ensure that your chiropractor is trained to work with pregnant patients.

Can I get a massage? Yes. Body massages are safe; however, avoid those that use excessive heating elements. Ensure the massage therapist is trained in performing prenatal massages.

Can I eat fish? It depends on the type of fish. Fish with high levels of mercury should be avoided and this includes king mackerel, shark, and swordfish. Mecury can cause harmful effects to your baby. Canned light tuna can be consumed but albacore tuna should be limited to 6 ounces a week. Shellfish like shrimp and lobster have only low levels of mercury and can be safely consumed. However, raw conch that is consumed in some carribean countries (e.g conch salad or "scorch" conch in the Bahamas) should be avoided. Sushi and sashimi should be avoided as consuming raw fish increases the risk of exposure to parasite and bacteria. If you must eat sushi, eat variants that include only cooked fish.

APPENDIX B: MEDICATIONS IN PREGNANCY

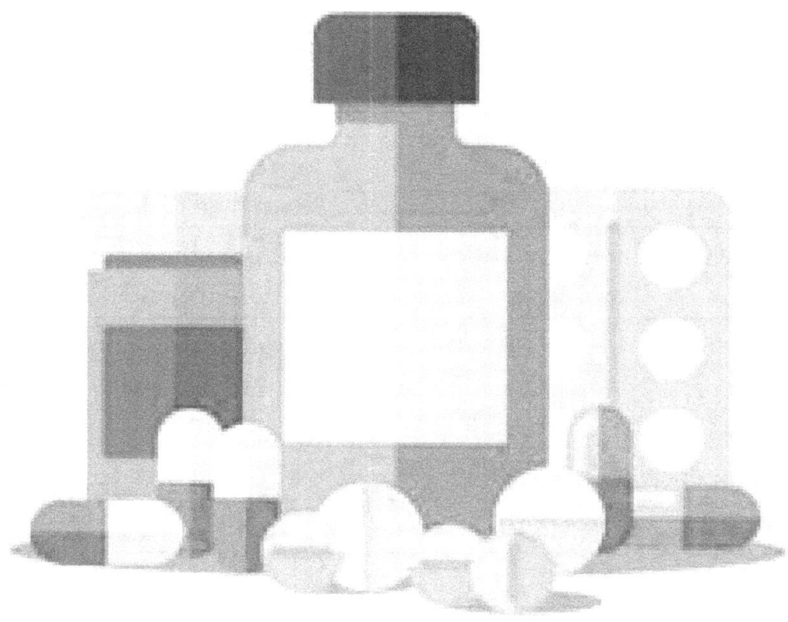

Before taking medications while pregnant, always consult your healthcare provider. Most medications should be avoided in the first trimester if possible, unless directed otherwise by your provider. The names in parentheses are examples of the brand name(s) that the medication may go by. This is listing is not complete.

Table 6

Name of Medication	Can It Be Used in Pregnancy?
Pain and Fever	
Paracetamol (Panadol®)	Yes
Paracetamol and Codeine (Panadeine®)	Yes
Metamizole sodium (Baralgin M®)	Yes
Ibuprofen (Motrin®, Advil®)	Yes, but not in third trimester
Naproxen sodium (Aleve®)	Yes, but not in the first and third trimesters
Aspirin (81 mg)	Only as prescribed by your physician and not in the third trimester.
Acetaminophen (Tylenol®)	Yes
Acetaminophen and Codeine	Yes
Cough, Cold, Allergy	
Guaifenesin (Mucinex®)	Yes, but not in first trimester
Dextromethorphan (Delsym®, Robitussin Cough®)	Yes
Dextromethorphan and Guaifenesin (Robitussin DM®, Histal DM®)	Yes
Phenylephrine	No
Pseudoephedrine	Yes, but not in first trimester
Oxymetazoline (Afrin® Nasal Spray)	No

Fexofenadine (Allegra®)	Yes
Loratadine (Claritin®)	Yes
Desloratadine (Clarinex®, Aerius®)	Yes
Diphenhydramine (Benadryl®)	Yes
Dimenhydrinate (Gravol®)	Yes
Cetirizine (Zyrtec®)	Yes
Zicam®	Yes
Antacids	
Ranitidine (Zantac®)	Yes
Omeprazole (Prilosec®, Alocid®)	Yes
Esomeprazole (Nexium®)	Yes
Pantoprazole (Pantecta®)	Yes
Maalox®, Mylanta®, Dica®, Tums®, Rolaids®	Yes
Bismuth subsalicylate (Pepto-Bismol®)	No
Nausea and Vomiting (Antiemetics)	
Doxylamine (Unisom® sleep tabs)	Yes
Dimenhydrinate (Gravol®, Unisom® sleep gels, Dramamine®)	Yes
Promethazine (Phenergan®)	Yes
Metoclopramide (Reglan®, Maxolon®)	Yes
Ondansetron (Zofran®)	Yes (Reserved for extreme cases of vomiting.)
Granisetron (Kytril®)	Yes (Reserved for extreme cases of vomiting.)

Antibiotics	
Penicillins: Amoxicillin, Ampicillin, Amoxicillin/Clavulanate (Augmentin®)	Yes
Macrolides: Erythromycin, Clarithromycin, Azithromycin	Yes
Tetracyclines: Doxycycline, Minocycline	No
Metronidazole (Flagyl®)	Yes, but not in first trimester
Metronidazole Vaginal Gel	Yes
Cephalosporins: Cephalexin (Keflex®), Ceftriaxone (Rocephin®), Ceftazidime (Fortum®), Cefuroxime (Zinacef®)	Yes
Aminoglycosides: Gentamicin, Tobramycin	No
Clindamycin	Yes
Antifungals	
Fluconazole (Diflucan®)	No
Clotrimazole (Canesten®, Gyne-Lotrimin®)	Yes
Miconazole (Monistat®)	Yes
Miconazole and Metronidazole (Gynotran®, Drez-V®)	Yes

www.ingramcontent.com/pod-product-compliance
Lightning Source LLC
Chambersburg PA
CBHW070758240726
48654CB00007B/118